Mo Rosser

SPORTS

APY

and practice

& Stoughton

THE HODDER HEADLINE GROUP

Acknowledgements

I am indebted to many friends and colleagues for their advice and support during the preparation of this book: to David Edge and Greta Couldridge for their guidance on content; to Heather Rosa for specialist advice on nutrition (chapter 4) and Dr Rosemary Jones for her expert advice on electric muscle stimulation (chapter 19); to the Swimming Pool and Allied Trades Association (SPATA) for information and photograph (page 261)

I thank my family for their enthusiasm and encouragement.
Finally, my grateful thanks to Llinos Davies who expertly edited the script with unfailing good humour and meticulous attention to detail.

This book is dedicated to our newborn grandson, Zachary William Rosser.

Orders: please contact Bookpoint Ltd, 130 Milton Park, Abingdon, Oxon OX14 4SB. Telephone: (44) 01235 827720, Fax: (44) 01235 400454. Lines are open from 9.00 - 6.00, Monday to Saturday, with a 24 hour message answering service. You can also order through our website: www.hodderheadline.co.uk

British Library Cataloguing in Publication Data
A catalogue record for this title is available from The British Library

ISBN 0 340 67320 6

First published 1997
Impression number   10 9 8 7
Year   2004 2003

Typeset by Wearset, Boldon, Tyne and Wear
Printed in Great Britain for Hodder & Stoughton Educational, a division of Hodder Headline, 338 Euston Road, London NW1 3BH by J. W. Arrowsmith Ltd., Bristol.

Contents

Introduction   vi

Part 1 General Principles   1
1 Ethical standards   2
    Legislation and codes of practice   2
    Personal safety and hygiene   5
    Safety factors to observe while exercising   8
2 The effects of exercise on body systems   13
    The organisational levels of the body   13
    The body's response to exercise   18
    The general benefits of exercise   24
3 The skeletal system   26
    The anatomical position   26
    The skeletal system   28
    Joints   41
    Skeletal muscle   50
    Energy for muscle contraction   56
4 Nutrition and diet   62
    Energy   62
    Carbohydrates   63
    Fats   66
    Proteins   68
    Vitamins   70
    Minerals   72
    Vitamin and mineral requirements of the athlete   73
    Chemicals which affect the body   74
    Water and other liquids   75

	Fibre	79
	Weight control	79
5	Physical principles relating to exercise	84
	Explanation of terminology	84
	Forces and their application	86
	Motion	88
	Gravity	92
	Levers	96
6	Concepts of movement	103
	Types of muscle work	103
	Range of movement	105
	The group action of muscles	106
	Analysis of muscle work for exercise schemes	108
	The classification of movement	111
	Part 2 Training for Fitness	114
7	Fitness training	115
	How to improve fitness	115
	The components of fitness	118
8	Cardio-respiratory endurance	120
	Improving cardio-respiratory endurance	120
	Muscle fitness	127
	Muscle strength	128
	Muscle endurance	136
	Plyometrics	137
	Strengthening exercises	138
	Speed	153
9	Flexibility and suppleness	157
	Factors which affect flexibility	157
	Methods of maintaining and increasing flexibility	159
	Stretching exercises	164
10	Rest and relaxation	176
	Rest	176
	Relaxation	176
11	Posture	183
	The effects of good and bad posture	183
	Evaluation of posture	185
	Corrective exercises for postural problems	190
12	Starting positions and exercise routines	201
	Starting positions	201
	Mobility exercises	205
	Warm up exercises	212
	Cool down exercises	213
	Breathing exercises	215
	Potentially damaging exercises	216

Part 3 Teaching exercises   228

13 The acquisition of skill   229
    Skill   229
    Motivation   232
    Planning exercise classes   234
    Types of aerobic classes   240
    Selecting music   241

14 Planning and assessment   244
    Planning   244
    Assessment   247

Part 4 Treatments   261

15 First Aid treatment   262
    Prevention of injury   262
    Immediate assessment of injury   263
    Immediate treatment   264
    Types of injury   268
    Treatment of soft tissue injuries   273
    Common injuries   275

16 Cryotherapy   286
    Methods of ice application   286
    Physiological effects of cooling the tissues   287
    Uses of cryotherapy   289
    Treatment   290
    Exercises following cryotherapy   293

17 Heat Therapy   295
    Methods of heat application   295
    General contra-indications to heat therapy   295
    Infra red treatment   296
    Steam treatments   307
    Sauna baths   311
    Spa pools/baths   315
    Paraffin wax   323

18 Mechanical massage   327
    Mechanical massage for sports therapy   327
    The gyratory vibrator   328
    Audio-sonic vibrator   333

19 Muscle stimulation   336
    Indications for use   336
    Terminology of muscle stimulation   337
    Nerve muscle physiology   337
    Muscle fibre types   342
    Electrical stimulation machines   344
    The stimulation of individual muscles   356

Further Reading   360
Index   361

Introduction

Sporting and fitness activities enhance our lives, providing us with challenge, satisfaction, pleasure, fun and sometimes frustration. Regular exercise helps to keep us young, fit and healthy and also protects us from developing many diseases. People are now very much aware of the great benefits to be derived from an active lifestyle, and increasing numbers of people participate in a wide variety of sporting or athletic activities. The number of leisure centres, gymnasiums, sports stadiums etc. is growing to meet this public demand.

All these centres require supervisory staff to ensure that they operate effectively and efficiently. Sports therapists have a very important role to play, as educators, advisors, trainers and instructors. They must become expert in their chosen field and be constantly aware that they are accountable for the instruction and advice they impart. They bear the responsibility for the well-being and safety of those in their care, and must therefore have sufficient knowledge to deliver safe and effective instruction and give accurate advice.

This book is an introduction to the field of sports therapy. It covers the basic theory of fitness and exercise, as well as the electrical modalities used in this field. It will enable the student to construct suitable programmes to meet the needs of differing clients.

It is impossible to cover all types of exercise in one book and further reading of specific training regimes is required.

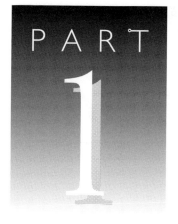

General Principles

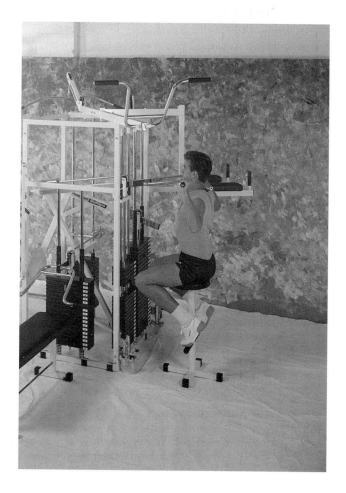

Ethical Standards

The highest standards of ethical conduct must be observed at all times. In addition to acquiring knowledge, understanding and expertise, therapists must consider their standard of behaviour in relation to colleagues, clients and others with whom they have contact. These factors will inspire confidence, establish a sound reputation and contribute to the success and satisfaction of your work.

Legislation and codes of practice

The sports therapist must be fully aware of all legislation related to their industry and must abide by these legal requirements. The following documents should be read and be available for reference at all times:

1 Code of Practice for Hygiene in the Clinic, and the Gymnasium.
2 Health and Safety at Work Act 1974
3 Consumer Protection Act 1987
4 Trade Descriptions Act 1968
5 Sale of Goods Act 1979
6 Local Government (Miscellaneous Provisions) Act 1976
7 Local Authority bye laws.

Adherence to these laws will ensure that the therapist practises in a professional and safe manner, for the benefit of the client and in the best interest of the clinic. The therapist's behaviour and standards of care, safety and hygiene reflect on the clinic as well as on the therapist. The following codes or practice should be used as a guide:

1 All treatments must be carried out safely, in accordance with legislative requirements.

2 The highest standards of hygiene must be adopted for the protection of the client, the therapist and other staff.

3 The services provided are efficient, of good quality and effective.

4 The time allocated and the cost of the treatment is appropriate and consistent.

5 The desired outcomes are established, and the treatment fully explained, discussed and agreed with the client. Accurate advice and information is given. This will promote clear understanding and gain client confidence.

6 The therapist will communicate efficiently and effectively with clients, colleagues, suppliers and others.

7 Consultation details are accurately, legibly and regularly recorded, and safely stored ensuring confidentiality at all times.

8 The procedures for health, safety and security are regularly monitored and immediate action taken if these do not meet with legislative requirements.

9 Qualified assistance is available to deal immediately with accidents or emergencies when the therapist requests it.

10 All personnel are promptly informed of any relevant changes in procedures and standards.

Relationships in the workplace

The therapist must develop a good working relationship with many different types of people. These may include colleagues, supervisors, managers, company representatives and salespeople. The ability to communicate politely and effectively with all of these people is very important. Always bear in mind the following points:

1 Speak politely, clearly, and courteously to everyone at all times.

2 Be respectful to those in authority, and be helpful to all colleagues, particularly to subordinates for whom you have responsibility.

3 Be loyal to your employer and colleagues; try to create a friendly working atmosphere.

4 Speak correctly at all times: do not use improper language. Consider the manner in which you answer or speak on the telephone; be clear, precise and polite.

5 Ask for help or advice politely, and give assistance willingly.

6 Discuss and resolve any problems or difficulties promptly, explaining your viewpoint courteously. Do not be argumentative or confrontational.

7 Respond promptly and clearly to all forms of communication, whether oral, written or non-verbal. Make sure that you understand and are understood by all concerned.

8 Be discreet and refrain from gossip. Do not repeat information given to you in confidence.

9 Take your responsibilities seriously; be honest and reliable at all times.

10 Be punctual and well organised. Aim to establish a sound reputation for high standards and efficient service.

Relationship with clients

Establishing a relationship with clients is extremely important. The therapist will deal with many different types of clients, and must adapt to a variety of personalities and problems. Clients may be young, old, confident, nervous, shy, apprehensive, pleasant, demanding, thin, slim, obese; they may have prior knowledge of the treatments or may require detailed explanations and advice. The therapist must be aware of these differences and react accordingly. Good rapport is essential to gain the clients confidence, and the following points should help to establish this.

1 Greet the client in a friendly, courteous and smiling manner.

2 Call the client by their name, as this creates an instant feeling of security. The surname can be used at first, progressing to first names as rapport develops.

3 Try to assess the type of client and how best to deal with them; note verbal and non-verbal signs. Do they have a confident air, or are there signs of shyness and hesitancy? Different types of people will require a different approach; learn to adapt to people and situations.

4 Speak clearly and politely, to make the client feel at ease.

5 Make the client comfortable and carry out a thorough consultation. Establish the client's desired outcomes and consider whether these are realistic and achievable. Ensure the client's privacy at all times.

6 Give accurate advice on suitable treatments, exercise programmes, etc. Discuss timings and cost, and make sure that the client fully understands and agrees with the objectives, effects and time span of the treatment. Ensure that you have their commitment.

7 Should the client request an unsuitable treatment or exercise routine, be firm but tactful in explaining why it would not be appropriate, and offer an alternative, more effective programme.

8 Do your utmost to deliver the most effective treatment suited to the needs of the client. Ask how the client feels after each treatment. This feedback is important because you may need to adapt or change the treatment next time. It also enables you to compare the effects of different treatments. This builds up expertise in selecting the most effective treatments.

9 Give the client home advice at the end of each treatment.

10 Keep a detailed, legible record of the consultation, and file in the appropriate place or on a pc.

11 Be honest and reliable, as this will gain trust and a good reputation. Do not make false claims for treatments, but clearly explain the benefits.

12 Be discreet and refrain from gossip; remember that clients often reveal personal problems during consultation. These facts and all personal details must be treated with the utmost confidentiality, and must not be repeated to colleagues or friends.

13 Be punctual, keep appointments and do not cancel at the last minute.

Personal safety and hygiene

The therapist

1 A daily bath or shower will maintain a clean skin and remove stale sweat, dirt and grease.

2 The use of an antiperspirant after bathing will prevent excessive sweating and the odour of stale sweat.

3 Underwear and tights should be changed daily and washed thoroughly in soapy water, as they absorb body odours.

4 White short-sleeved overalls should be crisp and well

laundered. Clothing for exercise should be unrestrictive, absorbent, smart and easy to wash. A clean overall should be worn every other day. Therapists should not wear the uniform out of doors; outdoor clothing should be changed in a cloakroom to prevent micro-organisms being brought into the clinic.

5 Hair must be clean and worn short or tied back off the face.

6 Teeth must be cleaned regularly, and a mouth wash can be used twice a day after eating. Smoking or spicy foods should be avoided. Regular dental checks are necessary to prevent the build-up of plaque.

7 Hands should receive particular care:
- they should be washed frequently before and after treatments, after handling any contaminated equipment, and using the toilet
- a bactericidal soap should be used
- a good hand cream should be applied nightly to keep skin soft and in good condition
- always wear rubber gloves when dealing with blood spills or disinfectants.

8 Nails should be kept short, well manicured and spotlessly clean, as micro-organisms can be harboured under the nail. Any nail enamel should be subtle and immaculate: well-buffed nails look more natural, and any dirt under the nail plate can be quickly seen and removed.

9 Feet should be well cared for:
- they should be washed and dried thoroughly at least once a day
- talcum or foot powder should be used
- nails must be cut regularly straight across
- well fitting flat shoes without holes and peeptoes will protect the feet and avoid pressure points
- appropriate well manufactured shoes must be worn for exercise (see advice to clients).

10 Therapists with colds or any throat infections should not treat clients if possible, but wearing a surgical mask will greatly reduce the likelihood of cross infection. Any infections of the hands or nails should be treated and covered with plaster and finger stalls; the therapist should not work if there are large areas of infection.

11 Food and drink should not be consumed or stored in the clinic, gymnasium or any working area (contamination could be transferred to the food and then to the mouth).

The client

1 Suitable clothing must be worn which will allow free unrestricted movement. Cotton is the best fabric as it allows easy absorption of perspiration. Cotton vests, T-shirts and shorts with elasticated waists or cotton bodies are all suitable. Some athletes wear track suits and leg warmers to maintain and raise body temperature during the warm up and stretch routines.

2 Footwear should be chosen with care to suit the activity; well constructed shoes should be bought from a reputable manufacturer. Footwear for exercise should be light, comfortable and offer good lateral support. The toe box should have sufficient height and length to prevent toes rubbing. The inner sole should absorb shock and the outer sole should be pliable, durable and non-slip. The tongue should be padded to protect the dorsum of the foot and the heel tab should not be too high or press on the heel. Socks alone should never be used for exercise because of the danger of slipping.

3 Hair should be tied back off the face, but hair combs, slides and pins should be avoided.

4 Jewellery should be removed.

5 Check for contra-indications, and seek doctor's advice if in doubt.

6 Do not allow exercise after a heavy meal or if under the influence of alcohol. Allow at least two hours after eating.

7 Do not allow exercise if pain killing drugs have been taken.

8 Exercises must be clearly explained; precautions and potential hazards must be stressed.

9 All equipment to be used must be fully explained and demonstrated, highlighting its effect and safety factors.

10 Exercises or training must be specific to the individual. Each client must work at their own pace and level, they must not exceed their capability, and they should not be forced or made to compete with others.

11 The different levels of fitness and age ranges must always be carefully considered when giving group exercise. Individuals must rest when tired and maximum heart rate must not be exceeded.

12 Exercises should not cause pain – if pain is experienced, stop exercising.

13 Select safe, stable starting positions.

14 Maintain good posture and body alignment when performing all the exercises, to prevent stresses and strains (see Chapter 11).

15 Practise correct breathing patterns; do not hold the breath.

16 Do not exercise cold muscles. Perform a thorough warm up lasting 10–15 minutes to include the large muscle groups. Warming tissues with various forms of heat therapy and massage will help, but is not enough; warm up exercises must be done as they allow the body systems to build up gradually, ready to meet the demand placed on them. Stretch carefully, slowly and smoothly, include all main joints, then perform the main activity. Perform cool down (warm down). Stretch again, finish with relaxation and deep breathing.

17 Shower and change clothing after exercise.

Remember:

- Do not exercise or stretch cold muscles.
- Always practise warm up exercises. If you arrive late for a class, perform a warm up at the side before joining in.

Safety factors to observe while exercising

The premises

- The room should be warm, well ventilated and without draughts.
- There must be good, even lighting with no pools of light or dark corners.
- Lights should be shielded with guards, particularly if games are played.
- The floor should be firm, smooth and non-slip and preferably sprung.
- There must be sufficient space for everyone to move freely with no overcrowding.
- The room should be clean and uncluttered. All apparatus not in use should be stored neatly away from the working area.
- Apparatus should be in good condition. There should be no rough edges or sharp protruding parts which could cause injury.

- There must be a sufficient number of well marked fire exits.
- A well stocked first aid box should be clearly visible and accessible.
- Shower and toilet facilities should be available.
- Water and fluids must be kept away from the working area as spillages make the floor slippery and dangerous.
- There should be no eating or drinking in the working area.
- Exercises should be supervised by qualified instructors at all times.
- Protective mats should be available for floor exercises.
- Mirrors should be available to check body alignment and correct performance of activities.

Safety guidelines for clients

These can be displayed in the exercise room or fully explained to clients at the beginning of the course. All of the points listed on page 7 will contribute to the client's safety while exercising. Additional safety points are:

- If you are suffering from any illness, please report. Check with your doctor if exercising is suitable.
- Do not exercise if feeling tired and fatigued or if suffering from muscle soreness.
- Empty the bladder before exercise.
- Take your pulse rate at regular intervals and do not exceed the maximum heart rate for your age.
- Keep to a few repetitions at the beginning of the course and add 3–5 with each session.
- Learn to perform the exercises carefully and correctly; pay attention to detail. Do not exercise half heartedly, mechanically or without concentration. Movements should be smooth and co-ordinated.
- Stretch carefully, smoothly and slowly; feel the stretch in the belly of the muscle and not at the tendon ends. Hold the stretch and release slowly.
- Do not bounce at the end of the range of movement or rapidly stretch muscles. This type of ballistic movement works against the stretch reflex and may result in small tears within the muscle.
- Breathe freely during exercise; do not hold the breath when stretching, but exhale as you move into the stretch.
- Maintain good body alignment (posture) while

exercising. Avoid strain on vulnerable areas such as neck, lower back and knees.

- If injury occurs, stop exercising immediately. Follow the RICED principle to deal with injury – Rest, Ice, Compression, Elevation and Diagnosis.
- Drink water during and at the end of the session to maintain fluid levels.

Safety when using equipment

- Buy equipment from a reputable dealer.
- Ask for a demonstration and try it before you buy.
- Make sure that it is regularly maintained according to the manufacturer's instructions.
- Follow the manufacturer's instructions for use.
- Use equipment for its intended purpose only.
- Check before use, ensuring that all parts are secure and that it is in good working order.
- Keep equipment clean, store it neatly and safely after use.
- Prepare and check all equipment before the exercise session starts.
- Any items for later use must be placed in a safe position, away from the working area.
- Do not allow clients to use equipment unsupervised; remember that you are responsible for their safety. You could be sued for negligence if an accident was to happen.
- Any equipment that is unstable, unsafe or too old must be removed from the clinic or gymnasium and clearly labelled 'Out of Order, Do Not Touch'.
- All electrical equipment must be regularly serviced and maintained in good working order. It must be checked before application to the client. Leads, insulation, plugs, terminals must be sound and secure; leads must not trail across the working area.
- Replace fuses when required with those of the correct rating. Do not overload the circuit with use of multiblocks.
- Machines must always be stable or placed on a stable base.
- Electrical equipment should not be placed near water or handled with wet hands.
- Keep machines clean and cover when not in use.

Contra-indications to exercise

All clients should have a thorough consultation before embarking on an exercise programme (see Chapter 14). Any of the following conditions would indicate that the client should not exercise, and if in doubt, always seek medical advice. Ensure that the client signs a consent form prior to treatment or exercise.

Common contra-indications are:

- *Recent injuries,* including fractures, strains, sprains, ruptures or tears. It is sometimes desirable to maintain fitness in other parts of the body while the injured part is immobilised. The exercises for other body parts must be carefully planned and performed, ensuring that no stress is placed on the injured part and surrounding tissues.
- *Heart conditions* – any history of heart disease. Appropriate exercise regimes are undertaken following heart attacks and surgery but these should be medically directed or supervised.
- *High blood pressure.* Exercise is generally allowed, if the blood pressure is controlled by drugs, but you should check with a doctor. Relaxation can help hypertensive clients but isometrics should never be performed.
- *Acute fevers* such as influenza, glandular fever, common colds, etc.
- *Infections* such as throat infections, measles, chicken pox, etc.
- *Inflammatory joint conditions* such as arthritis.
- *Neurological disorders* such as strokes, multiple sclerosis, etc. Exercises for these conditions must be medically supervised.
- *Undiagnosed illness* – seek a doctor's advice.
- *Musculo-skeletal* problems such as joint or back pain.
- Suffering from *pain* and *soreness in muscles.*
- During *pregnancy* or within 3 months of pregnancy. Gentle exercises only should be given during the first months of pregnancy; these anti-natal exercises should be medically supervised.
- After eating a heavy meal or under the influence of alcohol.
- If overtired, exhausted.
- If under the influence of pain killing drugs.
- If there has been any past difficulty with exercise.

Be particularly aware of the increase of potential health problems as the body ages. To be safe, people aged over 40 should have a medical check up before starting an exercise programme. Those who are at greatest risk are:

- the obese
- those with a history of heart problems in the immediate family
- hypertensives
- diabetics – doctor referral is important, especially if on insulin
- history of lung problems such as asthma, bronchitis, emphysema
- smokers
- refer these for a check up before commencing exercise programmes.

Questions

1 Explain briefly why the sports therapist must observe high standards of ethical conduct.
2 List six factors which contribute to safe practice.
3 Explain briefly how you would ensure a good working relationship with your working colleagues.
4 Explain briefly how you would make a client feel at ease, when visiting the clinic.
5 Explain how you would deal with a client who requested an unsuitable treatment.

6 List six factors which contribute to personal hygiene.
7 Give one reason why outdoor clothing should not be worn in the clinic.
8 Explain how you would minimise the risk of cross infection if you were working while suffering from the following:
i   a cold
ii an infection around one finger nail.

CHAPTER 2

The Effects of Exercise on Body Systems

To understand the beneficial effects of exercise, it is necessary to consider how the body systems contribute to athletic performance. The sports therapist must therefore have a sound basic knowledge of anatomy and physiology.

- Anatomy is the study of the *structure* of the body
- Physiology is the study of the *functions* of the body.

The structure and function of each system are obviously inter-linked and designed to carry out a specific function. The balanced interaction of all the systems is vital for maintaining stability of the internal environment, known as *homeostasis*, and for the proper functioning of the body.

An in-depth study of these subjects is not within the scope of this book and the therapist should refer to specialist texts.

The organisational levels of the body

There are five organisational levels of the body:

Chemical → Cellular → Tissue → Organ → System

Each will now be considered.

Chemical

At the very basic level are the chemical elements which form the body mass and carry out the processes necessary for sustaining life. There are approximately 109 recognised elements; 26 of these are found in the human body.

Oxygen, hydrogen, carbon and nitrogen form the highest percentage, making up about 96% of body weight. Calcium and phosphorus make up around 2%. Twenty elements make up the remaining 2%, and are found in very low concentrations; examples of these trace elements are iron, sodium, potassium, chlorine and magnesium.

Elements may combine or bond together to form compounds; eg, a sodium atom may combine with a chlorine atom to form sodium chloride. Chemical reactions result in the forming or the breaking of bonds between atoms. They are involved in the building of body structures and in the functioning of life-sustaining processes.

Cells

The cells are the basic structural and functional units of the body, which carry out all activities which maintain life. The body is made up of billions of cells; all have a similar basic structure, but they change slightly to suit their function, eg, blood cells differ from fat cells.

Figure 2.1   *A typical cell*

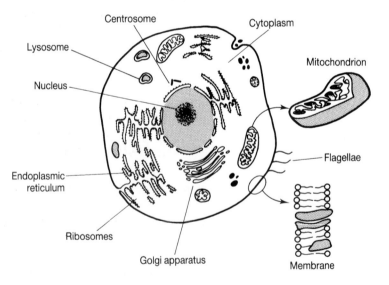

Cells require stable conditions in which to carry out their functions. The maintenance of stable conditions within the body is known as *homeostasis*.

Cells are bathed in extra-cellular fluid, which contains nutrients, gases and charged particles called ions. This fluid provides a medium for the transportation of substances in or out of the cell; the flow across the cell membrane will depend on the concentrations inside and outside the cells.

Muscle tissue cells are highly specialised as they have to release large amounts of energy for muscle contraction.

Tissues

The tissues of the body are groups of similar cells which work together to perform a specific function. All cells of one tissue will be the same, but the cells of different tissues will be modified to suit the function of that particular tissue. There are four main types of tissue in the body:

1 *Epithelial tissue:* this covers the body surfaces, lines the body organs and tubes, and forms glands.
2 *Connective tissue:* this supports and protects organs; it binds and connects tissues and organs together. There are many different types of connective tissue, each with a specific function:
    A *areolar* tissue is found under the skin and in between tissues
    B *adipose* tissue stores fat
    C *fibrous* tissue forms tendons and ligaments
    D *yellow elastic* tissue is found in organs where stretch and recoil are required, such as in the walls of arteries and bronchial tubes
    E *reticular* tissue forms a delicate network of support for cells in the spleen, liver and lymph nodes
    F *cartilage,* of which there are three types: hyaline which covers the ends of bones, fibro cartilage which forms intervertebral discs; and elastic cartilage forming the framework of the external ear
    G *blood* and *bone* tissue are also classified as connective tissue.
3 *Muscular tissue:* this includes smooth, cardiac, and skeletal muscle, and is able to contract and relax to product movement.
4 *Nervous tissue:* this co-ordinates the activities of the body as it initiates and transmits impulses. It is the communication system of the body.

Organs

Many tissues will be organised to form the organs of the body. Each organ has a specific function or functions to perform; eg, the stomach digests food, the lungs exchange gases, the heart pumps blood, the kidneys form urine and filter fluids, the ovaries produce and release ova. Organs form parts of the systems of the body.

Systems

Each body system consists of many organs which link together to perform a common function. All the systems are inter-related and function together to maintain life. There are 11 body systems.

These systems interact in a complex way to ensure that the body functions efficiently. During movement and exercise they all have an important role to play:

- Skeletal bones act as levers for movement.
- Joints allow for movement.
- Muscles contract to produce movement.
- The digestive system ingests, digests and absorbs nutrients which provide energy for muscle contraction and keep the body in good condition.
- The respiratory system takes in oxygen required by the energy producing muscle cells and eliminates the waste product carbon dioxide.
- The cardiovascular system transports nutrients and oxygen in the blood to the muscles to provide energy, and removes carbon dioxide and lactic acid from the muscles.
- The lymphatic system transports fat and removes waste.
- The nervous system initiates muscle contraction and co-ordinates movement.
- The pancreas (part of the endocrine system) secretes the hormones insulin and glucagon which regulate blood sugar levels.
- The skin plays a part in the regulation of body temperature through the production and evaporation of sweat. This is very important during intense exercise.
- The kidneys control the acid balance in the blood and retain substances that the body needs, such as glycogen.

Table 2.1   Systems of the body

System	Location	Function
Integumentary System	The skin and all its structures, nails, hair, sweat and oil glands	Protects, regulates temperature, eliminates waste. Makes Vitamin D, receives stimuli
Skeletal System	The bones, joints and cartilages	Supports, protects, aids movement, stores minerals, protects cells that produce blood cells
Muscular System	Usually refers to skeletal muscle but includes cardiac and smooth	Produces movement, maintains posture and produces heat
Nervous System	Brain, spinal cord, nerves, sense organs	Communicates and co-ordinates body functions
Cardio-Vascular System	heart, blood vessels, blood	Transports substances around body, helps regulate body temperature, prevents blood loss by blood clotting
Lymphatic System	Lymphatic vessels, nodes, lymph, spleen, tonsils and thymus gland	Returns proteins and plasma to blood. Carries fat from intestine to blood. Filters body fluid, forms white blood cells, protects against disease
Respiratory	Pharynx, larynx, trachea bronchi and lungs	Supplies oxygen and removes carbon dioxide
Digestive	Gastro-intestinal tract, salivary glands, gallbladder, liver and pancreas	Physical and chemical breakdown of food. Absorption of nutrients and elimination of waste
Urinary	Kidneys, ureters, bladder and urethra	Regulates chemical composition of blood. Helps to balance the acid/alkali content in the body, eliminates urine
Reproductive	Ovaries, testes etc.	Involved in reproduction
Endocrine	All the hormone producing glands	Regulates body activities through hormones

The body's response to exercise

The cardiovascular system: heart, blood and vessels

During exercise, contracting muscles require a steady supply of oxygen and nutrients for energy production, over and above the amount required for normal activities. The heart must beat harder and faster to meet this demand and as a result, it becomes stronger.

The heart and vessels respond and adapt in the following ways:

- The heart increases in size and volume.
- The heart pumps out more blood with each beat (stroke volume) and therefore pumps out more blood per minute (cardiac output).
- The heart pumps out more blood with each beat, so when the body is at rest, fewer beats per minute are necessary and the heart rate is lowered. Normal heart rate is around 72–76 beats per minute, but endurance athletes such as marathon runners may have heart rates as low as 40 beats per minute. This reduces the work load of the heart.
- There is an increase in capillary density to cardiac and skeletal muscles, which therefore increases blood supply.
- Blood vessels increase in size and number, and so blood flow is increased. This improves the delivery of oxygen and nutrients, and the removal of waste products.
- Increased levels of haemoglobin increase the oxygen carrying capacity of the blood.

Research has shown that regular aerobic activities will greatly improve heart function and endurance. Carefully graded and controlled exercises form part of cardiac rehabilitation following heart problems and heart attack.

The respiratory system: the respiratory tract and lungs

- During exercise there is an increase in the rate and depth of ventilation. The muscle's demand for more oxygen and the increase in the production of carbon dioxide stimulates deeper and faster breathing. During exercise, the volume of air breathed in and out of the lungs may be 30 times greater than when the body is at rest.

- The elasticity and condition of the lung tissue is improved.
- The blood supply to and from the lungs is increased.
- The condition of the muscles which move the thorax improves: the intercostals and diaphragm grow stronger as they are made to work harder.

Exercise and asthma

Asthma sufferers may exercise with caution but must not over-exert, as physical exertion can sometimes trigger an asthmatic attack. This is referred to as 'exercise induced asthma'. If breathing difficulties are experienced for longer than normal, ie, over five minutes, and there is obvious distress, medical advice should be sought quickly. Asthmatics should always have bronchodilators to hand.

Asthmatics derive benefit from exercise performed in short bursts with frequent rest intervals. It is better to exercise indoors than outdoors to avoid cold air, pollen and other allegens. Indoor swimming is ideal as it provides gentle exercise in a warm, humid atmosphere.

People who suffer from asthma should learn to recognise distress signals, and should take appropriate steps to control the condition. Research has shown that increased aerobic fitness can reduce the frequency of asthma attacks and allow asthmatics to exercise for longer periods.

Skeletal muscle

Muscle tissue responds to exercise in several ways, depending on the type of training and overload:

- Strength and bulk will improve in response to *resistance* exercises.
- Flexibility will improve with *stretch* exercises.
- Endurance will improve in response to *repetitive* exercises.

Strength and bulk

- Muscle strength will increase in response to sub-maximal or maximal overload. As the muscle strengthens, the load must be progressively increased.

- More motor units are recruited, which increases the strength of contraction.
- Muscle bulk (size) increase is mainly due to an increase in the contractile proteins actin and myosin.
- Bulk also increases because of an increase in the number of myofibrils. Research now indicates that the number of muscle fibres may also increase.
- Regular exercise results in an improvement in the energy producing systems and in the stores of the energy providing chemical compounds. Increased levels of adenosine triphosphate (ATP), phosphocreatine, enzymes and glycogen are found in muscle tissue.
- Generally males will bulk more readily than females. This is due to increased levels of the male hormone testosterone which is necessary for the synthesis of actin and myosin. Females show less bulking but will develop strength by progressive weight training. Some muscles bulk more readily than others; eg, biceps and quadriceps bulk readily while the abdominals do not.

Flexibility

Flexibility exercises will gently stretch musculotendinous components at a joint, and improve muscle elasticity and extensibility. Flexibility exercises at the end of an exercise programme will reduce muscle soreness (see Chapter 9).

Endurance

- Muscle endurance improves when a muscle is made to contract repeatedly against low or moderate resistance.
- Increase in the number and size of blood vessels to muscle fibres.
- Increase in capillary density to muscle fibres.
- Increase in blood flow, which increases the delivery of oxygen and removal of waste.
- Increase in the number of mitochondria in muscle cells, therefore increased efficiency in utilising oxygen for energy.
- Increase in glycogen stores. The increased availability of oxygen and glycogen raises the anaerobic threshold; as muscles use aerobic energy for longer periods, levels of lactic acid are reduced. Muscles can continue contracting for longer periods without fatigue.

Joints

The movement at joints stimulates the secretion of synovial fluid. This lubricates and nourishes the cartilage, thus improving its condition. This allows smoother movement at joints.

Stretching or full range flexibility exercises will maintain and increase the range of movement at joints. Joint range may be increased actively or passively:

1 *Active stretch* is a free movement performed by the client (see Chapter 9).
2 *Passive stretch* is performed by the therapist or partner applying pressure at the end of the range while the client's muscles are relaxed. This must be performed with great care and must only be undertaken after thorough training.

Connective tissue structures

The connective tissue structures around joints (the supporting ligaments, tendons and capsule) will improve in flexibility with regular exercise. The increased suppleness will reduce the likelihood of injury such as sprains, tears and ruptures.

Ageing and immobilisation result in a loss of flexibility. These groups benefit greatly from regular exercise to restore and maintain function, but every precaution must be taken not to over stress or strain.

Bones

Bones are strengthened in response to the stresses imposed upon them, particularly through exercise. More calcium and other minerals are deposited and more collagen is laid down, which improves the condition and strength of the bones. Exercise is particularly beneficial for post menopausal women, as exercise can delay and protect against the development of osteoporosis (a condition where bones become brittle and fracture easily due to a decrease in collagen and lack of mineral salts).

Metabolism

Exercise increases metabolic rate (the rate at which body activities use energy). An exercising muscle has a metabolic rate up to 50 times higher than a muscle at rest. It therefore expends 50 times more energy. The metabolic rate of skeletal muscle can vary to a greater degree than any other tissue.

Glycogen is the main source of fast energy, but when these stores are depleted or if the exercise is prolonged and of low/moderate intensity, then energy is obtained from fat (fatty acids and triglycerides). This fat is removed from fat stores all over the body.

Exercise increases muscle bulk and the body composition changes, with less fat but more muscle. It is an advantage to have a high proportion of muscle tissue as it has a high metabolic rate and utilises more energy than other tissues. Through regular exercise, low energy output can become high energy output. A regular aerobic programme and a controlled calorie diet will result in a reduction of body fat and lower blood cholesterol levels.

Neuromuscular co-ordination

Stimuli are initiated in the brain and transmitted via motor nerves to the muscles resulting in their contraction. This results in movement at the joints. The brain also co-ordinates the patterns of movement which result in skilled performance. Exercise increases the speed of neural response, and regular practice reinforces patterns of movement. Therefore co-ordination, speed, balance and rhythm improve and performance is enhanced.

The general benefits of exercise

Having studied the effects of exercise on the body, we can see why it is beneficial for general health and fitness. Research has shown that all age groups can derive some benefit through regular exercise, providing that the intensity is appropriate to fitness levels. In response to exercise, the body adapts to the stresses imposed upon it, which result in certain physiological changes. The extent of these changes will depend upon the amount and duration of the overload, and to which systems it is applied. Appropriate exercise regularly practised will improve physical fitness, promote health and reduce the risks of developing many diseases. The beneficial effects derived from exercise are both physiological and psychological.

Physiological benefits of exercise

1 Improvement in cardio-vascular function, ie, a stronger heart and improved circulation.
2 Improvement in respiratory function, ie, healthier and stronger lungs, deeper breathing.
3 Improvement in muscle tone, strength and stamina, power and speed.
4 Improvement in flexibility and tensile strength of tendons and ligaments. This will increase the range of movement at joints, movements will be easier and the likelihood of trauma (injury) reduced.
5 Improvement in the condition of joints. Exercise increases the production of synovial fluid which lubricates and nourishes the cartilage, resulting in smoother movements.
6 Improvement in bone density and strength. This is particularly important for women as it helps to combat osteoporosis.
7 Improvement in neuro-muscular co-ordination which improves rhythm, balance, timing and reaction time, and enhances skill levels. Activities become easier.
8 Reduction in fat reserves. As the proportion of muscle tissue increases, the metabolic rate will increase; this will increase demand for fuel and thus reduce fat stores.
9 Increased ability to utilise fat or fuel. As the oxygen intake increases, more is available for the aerobic breakdown of fat for fuel. Fat is predominantly used when the exercises are of low/moderate intensity and long duration.
10 Lowering of total blood cholesterol levels. Exercise lowers the 'bad' low density lipoproteins and raises the 'good' high density lipoproteins.
11 Reduction in trauma and pain due to improved muscle strength, flexibility and range of movement.

12 Reduction in the risk of developing debilitating diseases:
- hypertension (high blood pressure): exercise lowers blood pressure
- heart disease: the heart is strengthened by exercise
- blocked arteries and strokes: exercise causes the lowering of blood cholesterol and reduction of plaque formation
- diabetes: exercise lowers insulin levels
- cancer: exercise protects against certain forms of cancer.

Exercise also reduces stress levels, which is a contributory factor in many of these illnesses.

Psychological benefits of exercise

1 Feelings of well-being, achievement and euphoria.
2 An increase in self confidence and self worth.
3 Reduction in stress levels.
4 Promotion of relaxation and sleep.

To achieve these benefits, exercises must be carefully selected and performed accurately and regularly. Exercise should always be specific to the individual, and the degree of ease or difficulty should be appropriate to the level of fitness. Inappropriate exercises that are too difficult or are casually and excessively performed, can result in damage and pain. Training or practice must be regular, because, if training stops, the beneficial effects are quickly lost.

The damaging effects of inappropriate exercise are:

- Muscle strain, tears and soreness
- Ligamentous sprains, overstretching and tears
- Joint stresses
- Bone stresses
- Inflammation of tendons, bursae and joint capsules, namely tendonitis, bursitis and capsulitis
- All these traumas produce pain which adversely affects daily activities, relaxation and sleep. Pain may also produce feelings of tension, stress, depression, disappointment and low self esteem.

Questions

1 State four physiological benefits of exercises.
2 State four psychological benefits of exercises.
3 List six damaging effects of inappropriate exercises.
4 Explain briefly how heart function improves as a result of regular training.
5 State why the oxygen carrying capacity of the blood increases as a result of regular exercises.
6 Explain briefly why the volume of air breathed in and out of the lungs must increase during exercise.
7 State three effects of exercise on skeletal muscle.
8 Give reasons why suppleness increases as a result of regular exercises.
9 Explain briefly why exercise protects against the bone disease, osteoporosis.
10 Explain why it is advantageous to have high muscle tissue to low fat tissue ratio.

CHAPTER 3

The Skeletal System

This chapter deals with the structure and function of bones, cartilages and joints.

Bones form the framework of the body, giving it shape.

Cartilages protect the ends of bones and act as shock absorbers at joints.

When two or more bones meet, a joint is formed. As muscles contract, they pull on the bones, resulting in movement at the joint.

The anatomical position

Before we can describe body movement, we must have a basic position or static posture which is used as a common reference point for describing surfaces, relationships and directions of movement. This is known as the anatomical position.

In the anatomical position the body is upright, feet slightly apart with toes pointing forward. The arms hang to the sides with the palms of the hands facing forwards. (Note the difference to the normal standing position, when the palms of the hands face the sides of the body.)

With the body in this position the surfaces can be identified, and the direction of joint movement can be described in terms of planes and axes of movement.

Terminology

It is important to be familiar with the terms used to describe aspects of the body in the anatomical position, and also to describe the position of structures relative to each other.

Table 3.1 Terms used to describe the anatomical position

Surface or structure	Position
Anterior or ventral structure	a surface that faces forwards; a structure which is further forward than another
Posterior or dorsal	a surface that faces backwards; a structure which is further back than another
Medial	a surface or structure that is nearer the mid-line than another
Lateral	a surface or structure that is further away from the mid-line than another
Proximal	a structure that is nearer the root or origin, ie nearer the trunk
Distal	a structure that is further away from root or origin, ie, further away from the trunk
Superficial	a structure that is nearer the surface than others
Deep	a structure that lies beneath the others
Superior	a structure higher than others, ie towards the head
Inferior	a structure lower than others

The skeletal system

This is the bony framework of the body and is composed of:

- Bones
- Cartilages which cover the ends of articulating bones
- Joints or articulations (where two or more bones meet).

The functions of the skeletal system

- Support – the bony framework gives shape to the body, supports the soft tissues and provides attachment for muscles.

Figure 3.1 *The skeletal system (a) anterior view (b) lateral view*

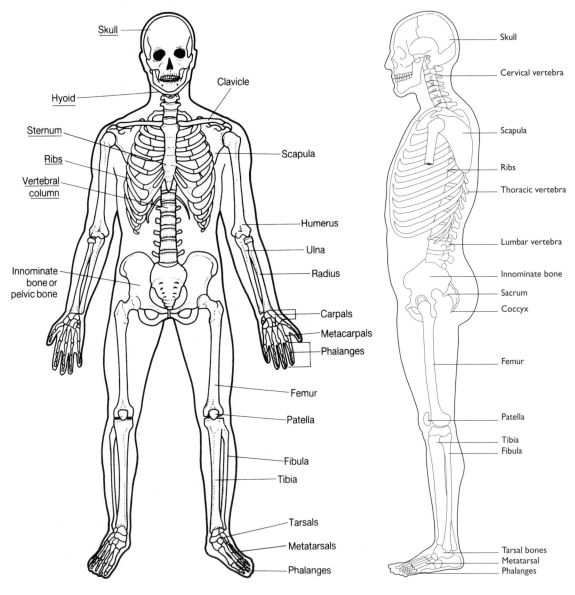

(a)

(b)

- Protection – the bony framework protects delicate internal organs from injury; eg the brain is protected by the skull; the heart and lungs are protected by the rib cage.
- Movement – this is produced by a system of bones, joints and muscles. The bones act as levers, and muscles pull on the bones, resulting in movement at joints.
- Storage of minerals – bones store many minerals, particularly calcium and phosphorus.
- Storage of energy – fats or lipids stored in the yellow bone marrow are broken down and used by the body when required.
- Storage of tissue which forms blood cells – special connective tissue called red bone marrow produces blood cells. Red bone marrow is found in the spongy bone of the pelvis, vertebrae, ribs, sternum, skull and the ends of the femur and humerus.

The structure of bone

Bone is a very hard connective tissue consisting of cells, collagen fibres and a matrix or ground substance. The matrix is impregnated with mineral salts such as calcium carbonate and calcium phosphate. As these salts are laid down, the tissue calcifies and hardens. Bone is a flexible living tissue and has the capacity to repair if damaged. There are two types of bone tissue:

1 *Compact* bone is a hard dense tissue which forms the outer layer of bones and gives them strength.
2 *Cancellous* bone forms the inner mass of bone. The spongy structure makes bones lighter.

Bones are enclosed in a dense layer of fibrous connective tissue known as the *periosteum*. This layer contains blood vessels which deliver nutrients to the bone, nerve and bone cells. Tendons (which attach muscles to bone) and ligaments (which join bones together) blend with the periosteum.

There are different types of *bone cells*, which are found in the periosteum or scattered throughout compact and spongy bone. They include:

- *Osteoblasts*: the bone builders, which produce minerals and collagen needed for strong bones
- *Osteocytes*: the main cells of bone tissue, which carry out the activities necessary for maintaining healthy bones

■ *Osteoclasts*: the bone clearers, which absorb and remove bone.

Exercise strengthens bones because they adapt to stress by laying down more calcium and other minerals, and also by increasing collagen fibres.

Fractures and other injuries to bones may occur in sports, and other physical activities. These must be quickly diagnosed and fixed to limit damage. An adequate length of time must be allowed for the fracture to heal.

Types of bones

There are four different types of bones, named according to their shape.

■ Long bones are longer than their width, eg: femur, tibia, fibula, humerus, radius, ulna, metacarpals, phalanges.
■ Short bones are of almost equal width and length, eg: carpal and tarsal bones.
■ Flat bones are flat thin bones, found where protection is needed and also where a broad surface is required for the attachment of muscles, eg: skull bones, scapulae, sternum, ribs.
■ Irregular bones are all the bones with complex shapes that do not fit into the above categories, eg: vertebrae, sacrum, innominate bone, sphenoid, ethmoid.

Other small bones found in the body but not named according to shape, are called sesamoid bones: small rounded bones that develop within tendons. They enable the tendon to move smoothly over the underlying bone, eg: the patella.

The bones of the skeletal system

It is difficult to study and visualise bones by simply using diagrams. The work is easier to learn and is made much more interesting when a model skeleton and model bones are used. These can be examined, the important features identified and related to one's own body. Only the important and relevant features have been included in the following text. However, remember to identify the features on model bones and palpate (feel) on your own body where possible.

The human skeleton is made up of 206 bones, which are grouped into two main divisions:

■ the *axial* skeleton forms the core or axis of the body
■ the *appendicular* skeleton forms the girdles and limbs.

The axial skeleton

The bones of the axial skeleton include the:

1 Skull (head)
2 Vertebral column (spine)
3 Sternum (breast bone)
4 Ribs
5 Hyoid bone (small bone in neck below mandible).

The appendicular skeleton

The bones of the appendicular skeleton include upper limb bones and lower limb bones.

Table 3.2   The bones of the appendicular skeleton

Upper limb bones	Lower limb bones
Clavicle (collar bone)	The innominate or pelvic bone (hip bone)
Scapula (shoulder blade)	Femur (thigh bone)
Humerus (upper arm bone)	Patella (knee cap)
Radius (forearm – lateral)	Tibia (large bone of lower leg – medial)
Ulna (forearm – medial)	Fibula (thin bone of lower leg – lateral)
Carpals (wrist)	Tarsals (ankle)
Metacarpals (palm)	Metatarsals (foot)
Phalanges (fingers)	Phalanges (toes)

Features of the skeletal bones

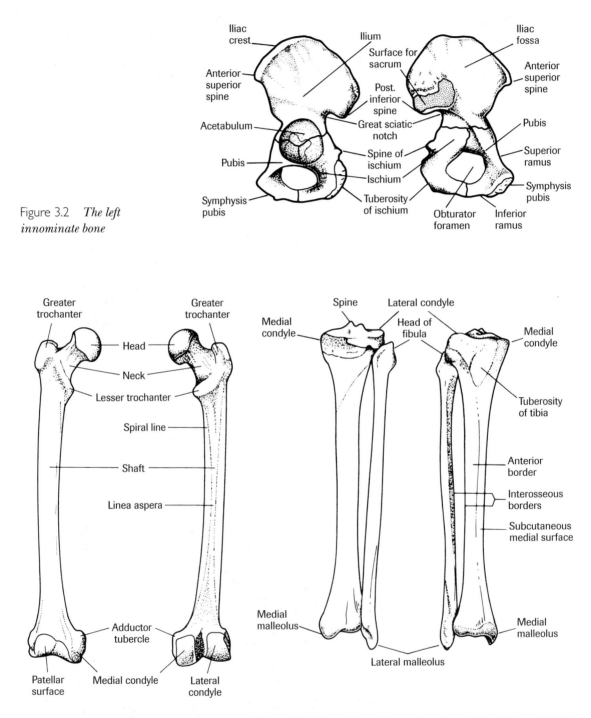

Figure 3.2 *The left innominate bone*

Figure 3.3 *Anterior and posterior views of the right femur*

Figure 3.4 *Posterior and anterior views of the tibia and fibula*

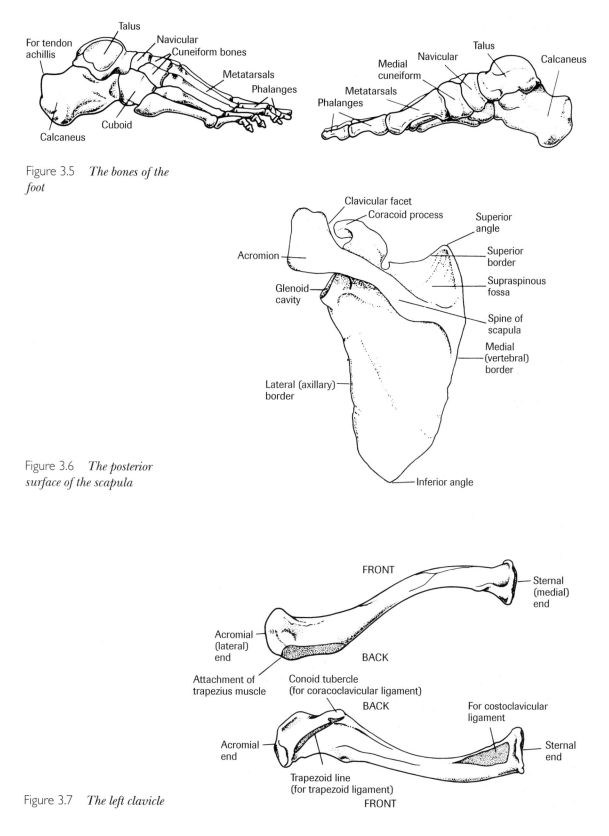

Figure 3.5   *The bones of the foot*

Figure 3.6   *The posterior surface of the scapula*

Figure 3.7   *The left clavicle*

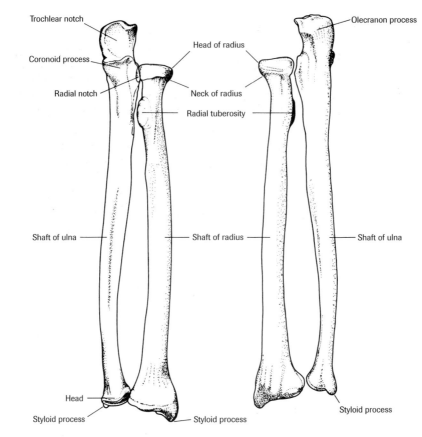

Figure 3.8   *The left radius and ulna*

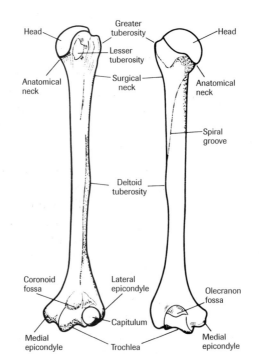

Figure 3.9   *The left humerus*

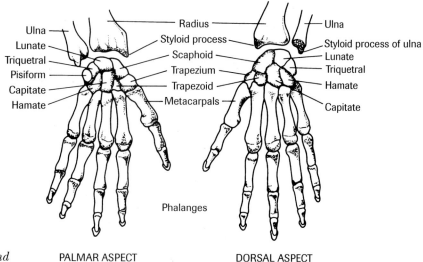

Figure 3.10   *The left hand*   PALMAR ASPECT   DORSAL ASPECT

The vertebral column (spinal column)

The vertebral column is composed of 33 vertebrae. Some are fused together making 26 bones.

The column is divided into five regions:

- Cervical – 7 vertebrae (neck)
- Thoracic – 12 vertebrae (upper back)
- Lumbar – 5 vertebrae (lower, small of back)
- Sacral – 5 fused vertebrae (sacrum)
- Coccygeal – 4 fused vertebrae (coccyx)

The vertebrae are separated by inter vertebral discs of fibro cartilage. The vertebrae and discs are bound together by strong powerful ligaments. There is very little movement between adjacent vertebrae, but the total combined movement along the whole length allows considerable movement of the trunk.

The movements of the vertebral column are:

- flexion
- extension
- side flexion
- rotation.

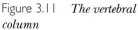

Figure 3.11   *The vertebral column*

There is a greater range of movement in the cervical and lumbar regions than in the thoracic. These variations are due to the length and direction of the spinous processes, the ratio between the height of the discs and the height of the vertebral body, and to the tension of the supporting ligaments.

Flexion and extension of the neck occur in the cervical region. Flexion and extension of the trunk occur mainly in the lumbar region. Rotation of the trunk occurs mainly in the thoracic region.

All vertebrae except the 1st and 2nd cervical (atlas and axis) have certain features in common but they vary in size, becoming larger lower down for weight bearing. The column is not straight but has curves along its length.

Curves of the vertebral column

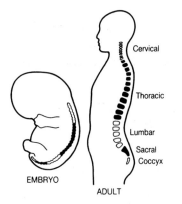

Figure 3.12   *Vertebral curves in the embryo and adult*

The vertebral column shows curves along its length. These are seen in the cervical, thoracic, lumbar and sacral regions. The thoracic and sacral curves are primary curves, being present before birth. The cervical and lumbar curves are secondary curves and develop after birth. The cervical develops when the baby lifts its head, the lumber develops as the baby learns to sit and stand. When viewed posteriorly:

- the cervical curve is concave
- the thoracic curve is convex
- the lumbar curve is concave
- the sacral curve is convex.

Spinal problems

Certain spinal problems result in exaggerated or abnormal spinal curves. When viewed posteriorly the following curves may be seen:

- *Kyphosis* is an exaggerated *thoracic* curve with increased convexity and forward flexion.
- *Lordosis* is an exaggerated *lumbar* curve with increased concavity and extension.
- *Kypho-lordosis* is a combination of the above.
- *Scoliosis* is a *lateral deviation* of the spine. It may deviate to the right or to the left and may show a long C curve or an S curve.

These curves are accompanied by muscle imbalance; ie, some muscles will be too tight and the opposite groups will be overstretched. Appropriate exercises are required to correct these problems.

These problems are fully discussed in Chapter 11.

A typical vertebra

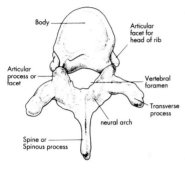

Figure 3.13   *A thoracic vertebra*

A typical vertebra is composed of several major parts: The main parts are:

1 The body: a mass of cancellous bone surrounded by compact bone. Body weight is transmitted through the vertebral bodies and inter-vertebral discs.
2 The neural or vertebral arch: a strong arch of bone enclosing the vertebral foramen. It protects the spinal cord which runs through the vertebral foramen.
3 The spinous process: projects backwards.
4 The transverse processes: project sideways. They provide attachment for many muscles and ligaments.
5 Four facets: articulating surfaces for the vertebrae above and below.

Nerves leave the spinal cord and pass through the inter-vertebral foramina between the vertebrae.

The inter-vertebral discs

These lie between the bodies of the vertebrae. They act as shock absorbers and allow for compression and distortion along the column. They are made up of the nucleus pulposus which is a jelly like material containing a high percentage (85%) of water. Surrounding this is the annulus fibrosus which is composed of many rings of elastic fibres woven at angles to each other. It is thus able to expand and move to absorb compression forces.

As we grow older the nucleus loses its water binding capacity, fibrocartilage replaces the gelatinous substance and the nucleus gradually hardens. The annulus fibrosus also loses its elasticity. As elasticity and flexibility is lost, the hardened rigid disc becomes more susceptible to injury. If the compression forces are abnormally strong or sudden, the annulus fibrosus may tear or rupture and the nucleus protrudes and pushes into the space. This is known as a 'slipped disc' or disc prolapse. If this protrusion presses against a nerve as it passes out of the spinal canal through the inter-vertebral foramen, then neurological symptoms will be felt along the path of the nerve, ie, pain, tingling, pins and needles, numbness etc.

Disc problems can occur at any time but the likelihood increases as we get older. It is therefore extremely important to consider the age and medical condition of clients when giving any neck and trunk exercises. Failure to do so can result in very serious injury.

Dangerous movements

The most hazardous movement is trunk forward flexion as this movement takes place mainly in the lumbar spine. About 20 per cent of the movement occurs between the fourth and fifth lumbar vertebrae, and 60 to 70 per cent occurs between the fifth lumbar and the first sacral vertebrae. There is therefore a high risk of damage in this area.

The body girdles

There are two girdles, the pelvic girdle and the shoulder girdle.

The pelvic girdle (or pelvis)

This is the circle of bone commonly called the hips. It protects various organs, eg, the uterus and bladder, and it transmits body weight to the legs. It is shaped rather like a basin and has an inner and outer surface.

The pelvic girdle is made up of three bones – two innominate bones and the sacrum (part of the vertebral column).

The two large innominate or pelvic bones articulate in front at a cartilagenous joint called the 'pubic symphysis', at the back they articulate on each side of the sacrum at gliding synovial joints called the 'sacro-iliac joints'. There is hardly any movement at these joints as they fit tightly together and are held in place by very strong ligaments.

The shoulder girdle (the pectoral girdle)

The shoulder girdle is composed of 2 clavicles in front and 2 scapulae at the back. Anteriorly each clavicle articulates with the sternum at the sterno-clavicular joint. Laterally the clavicles articulate with the acromion process of the scapula

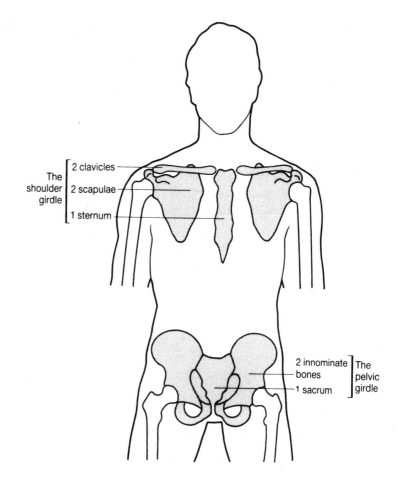

Figure 3.14 *Shoulder and pelvic girdles*

at the acromio-clavicular joint. The girdle joins the upper limbs to the axial skeleton.

The shoulder girdle forms an incomplete ring of bone around the upper thorax joined by muscles at the back. This arrangement allows for a wide range of movement both of the shoulder girdle and the shoulder joint.

The thoracic cavity

This is the bony cage of the chest, composed of the sternum, the 24 ribs and the 12 thoracic vertebrae.

The sternum

The sternum or breast bone is a flat narrow bone made up of three parts:

■ the manubrium: top part, squarish in shape

■ the body: long middle part
■ the xiphoid process: the small pointed lower end.

The ribs

The ribs are narrow flat bones, articulating with the thoracic vertebrae behind and to the sternum in front. The ribs are arranged in pairs one on the right and the other on the left.

■ Seven pairs are true ribs, which join the sternum
■ Five pairs are false ribs, which join the rib above. Two of these are called floating ribs as they have no attachment in front.

The ribs are joined to the sternum or to each other by a strip of hyaline cartilage, called the costal cartilages.

Small muscles known as the 'intercostal muscles' fill the spaces between the ribs. They lie in two layers; the eleven internal intercostals and the eleven external intercostals on each side of the chest. A large muscle called the 'diaphragm' forms the floor of the thoracic cavity. The lungs lie within and are protected by the thoracic cavity.

The mechanism of breathing

During breathing, the capacity of the thorax must increase so that air can be taken in and then must decrease so that air can be forced out. *Inspiration* is breathing in, *expiration* is breathing out. During inspiration, the intercostal muscles contract and swing the ribs upwards and outwards; the sternum is pushed forwards, and the diaphragm moves downwards. Thus the capacity of the thorax increases sideways, forwards and downwards and the pressure inside the thorax is lowered. When the pressure is reduced below atmospheric pressure (ie, air outside the body), air will rush in and fill the lungs. Oxygen passes into the blood stream through the walls of the capillaries surrounding the lungs and carbon dioxide passes the other way. During expiration the intercostal muscles relax, the diaphragm moves upwards, the ribs and sternum collapse back and the lungs recoil. This increases the pressure in the lungs and air is forced out.

During exercise, more oxygen is required to produce energy for muscle contraction. Therefore the intercostals and diaphragm work harder and as a result improve in strength and condition. The elasticity and condition of the lungs improves in the same way.

Questions

1 Compare the two main divisions of the human skeleton.
2 List the bones in each division.
3 Explain the functions of the skeletal system.
4 Explain why cancellous bone is sometimes known as spongy bone.
5 List the four main types of bones and give one example of each.
6 Describe the anatomical position.
7 Define the following terms: anterior surface, proximal end, medial, superior structure, deep muscle.

8 Name the regions of the vertebral column and give the number of vertebrae in each.
9 Give two functions of the inter-vertebral discs.
10 Compare the following spinal problems: Kyphosis, Lordosis and Scoiolsis.
11 List the bones that form the thoracic cavity or thorax.
12 Where may the xiphoid process be located?
13 Explain the terms: true and false ribs.

Joints

When two or more bones meet they form a joint, sometimes called an articulation. All body movement occurs at joints, from the small movements of the fingers to the large movements of the shoulder. The bones are held together by connective tissue and are moved by the contraction of skeletal muscle.

The shape of the articulating bones and the flexibility and tensile strength of the surrounding connective tissue determines the strength, stability and movement of joints.

Bones with curved surfaces that fit into each other and are close together form strong stable joints with less movement. Bones with little curvature that fit loosely are less stable but allow greater movement.

Terminology of joint movement

The following terms are used to describe the direction of joint movement.

- *Flexion* – the bringing together of two surfaces (a bending movement) eg, bending the elbow or knee.
- *Extension* – movement in the opposite direction (a straightening movement) eg, straightening the elbow or knee.

- *Abduction* – movement away from mid line, eg taking the arm away from the body.
- *Adduction* – movement towards mid line, eg taking the arm back to the body adding.
- *Rotation* – movement around a long axis, which may be medial rotation or lateral rotation, eg turning the arm in or turning the arm out.
- *Circumduction* – movement where the limb describes a cone whose apex lies in the joint. A combination of flexion, abduction, extension and adduction, eg, circling the shoulder or hip round and round.
- *Pronation* and *supination* are movements that occur between the radius and ulna: supination turns the hand forwards or upwards; pronation turns the hand backwards or downwards.
- Movements of the ankle joint: *Dorsi-flexion* – pulling the foot upwards; *Plantar flexion* – pointing the foot downwards (these occur at the ankle joint).
- Movements of the foot: *inversion* – turning the sole of the foot inwards; *eversion* – turning the sole of the foot outwards (these occur between the tarsal joints).
- Movements of the shoulder girdle (and jaw): *elevation* – lifting the shoulder (jaw) upwards; *depression* – dropping the shoulders (jaw); *protraction* – drawing the shoulders (jaw) forward; *retraction* – drawing the shoulders (jaw) backwards.
- Movements of the head and trunk: *forward flexion* – bending head or trunk forward; *side flexion* – bending head or trunk to the side (it may be right side flexion or left side flexion); *extension* – moving the head or trunk backwards; *rotation* – turning the head or trunk to the right or to the left a twisting movement; *circumduction* – moving the head or trunk in a circular motion.

Some joints only move in two directions, eg the elbow and knee, while others will move in six directions, eg, the shoulder and hip joints. Some muscles will be flexors, producing flexion at the joint, while other muscles will be extensors, producing extension at the joint and so on. When one group of muscles contracts to produce movement (the agonists) the opposite groups must relax to allow the movement to take place (the antagonists). See Chapter 6.

Body planes

These are imaginary surfaces along which movements take place. There are *three* planes, which lie at right angles to each other:

- *Sagittal Plane* (lies parallel with the sagittal suture of the skull). This plane divides the body into right and left parts. Flexion and extension movement are in this plane.
- *Coronal or Frontal Plane* (parallel with the coronal suture of the skull). This plane divides the body into front and back. Abduction and adduction movements are in this plane.
- *Horizontal or Transverse Plane* (parallel with a flat floor). This plane divides the body into upper and lower parts. Rotational movements are in this plane.

Axes

The axis of movement is a line around which movement takes place (in the same way as the earth revolves around its axis). It is always at right angles to the plane of movement.
There are three axes of movement:

- *sagittal* – from back to front (imagine a rod passing from front to back).
- *coronal/frontal* – from side to side (imagine a rod passing from side to side)
- *vertical* – straight up and down (differs from plane, imagine a rod vertical to the floor)

Examples of the planes and axes of certain movements when the body is in the anatomical position:

- Flexion and extension of the elbow is in a sagittal plane with frontal axis.
- Abduction and adduction of the hip will be in a frontal plane and sagittal axis.
- Turning the head from right to left will be in a horizontal plane and vertical axis.

Try these movements and work out others and remember the movement must be in one of three planes and the axis will be at right angles to the plane.

Classification of joints

There are three main groups:

1 *Fibrous* – immovable joints. The bones fit tightly together and are held firmly by fibrous tissue. There is no joint cavity; examples are the sutures of the skull.

2 *Cartilaginous* – slightly movable joints. The bones are connected by a disc or fibro-cartilage. There is no joint cavity. Examples are the symphysis pubis (between the pubic bones) and the inter-vertebral joints (between the vertebral bodies).

3 *Synovial joints* – freely movable joints. These are the most numerous in the body. There are six different types of synovial joints. They are classified according to their planes of movement, which depends on the shape of the articulating bones. All the freely movable joints of the body are synovial joints and although their shape and movements vary, they all have certain characteristics in common.

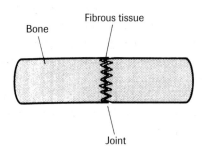

Figure 3.15   *A fibrous joint*

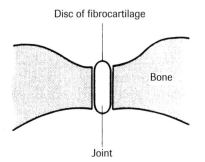

Figure 3.16   *A cartilaginous joint*

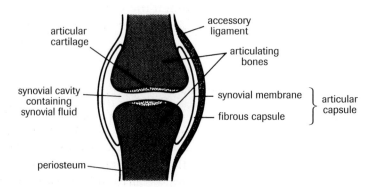

Figure 3.17   *A synovial joint*

Features of a typical synovial joint

- A joint cavity (space within the joint).
- The synovial membrane lining the capsule which produces synovial fluid.
- Synovial fluid or synovium; a viscous fluid which lubricates and nourishes the joint. Regular exercise stimulates an increase in the production of synovial fluid, therefore lubrication and nourishment of the cartilage is increased.
- Hyaline cartilage which covers the surfaces of the articulating bones. It is sometimes called articular cartilage, it reduces friction and allows smooth movement. With age, injury or disease there may be erosion or damage of this cartilage. Friction will increase as bone moves over bone, and the joint will be stiff and movements painful. Regular exercise with the increased lubrication will delay the onset of these problems but if there is joint damage, exercises must only be performed under medical supervision.
- Capsule or articulating capsule; this surrounds the joints like a sleeve. It holds the bones together and encloses the cavity. The capsule is strengthened on the outside by ligaments which help to stabilise and strengthen the joints. Ligaments may also be found inside a joint holding bones together increasing stability. The movement at any joint will be governed by the tightness or rigidity of the capsule and ligaments. Flexibility exercises and full range mobility exercises will maintain and increase the extensibility of these structures and maintain full range joint movement.

DISCS (MENISCI)

Some joints have pads of fibro-cartilage called *discs*. They are attached to the bones and give the joint a better 'fit'; they also cushion movement, eg, cartilages of the knee. These structures are prone to damage and tearing usually as a result of excessive stress and rotational forces.

BURSAE

Any movement produces friction between the moving parts. In order to reduce friction, sac-like structures containing synovial fluid are found between tissues. These are called *bursae* and are usually found between tendons and bone. These may become inflamed following injury or repetitive stress. This results in swelling, stiffness and pain of the joint.

Table 3.3   The six synovial joints

Type of joint	Examples	Movements
■ Gliding joints	Intercarpal and intertarsal joints.	Multiaxial movements limited to gliding or shifting.
■ Hinge joints	Elbow, ankle, interphalangeal joints (joints of fingers and toes). Uniaxial and one plane only – (sagittal plan, frontal axis).	Movements – flexion and extension
■ Pivot joints	Superior radio-ulnar joint and atlas axis (moves the head left to right). Uniaxial and one plane only (horizontal plane, vertical axis).	Movements – rotation
■ Ellipsoid (condyloid) joints	Wrist (radio-carpal), knuckle (metacarpo-phalangeal joint). Biaxial – in two planes (sagittal and frontal planes, frontal and saggital axes).	Movements – flexion, extension, adduction, abduction, circumduction
■ Saddle joints	Carpo-metacarpal joint or thumb (base of thumb). Multiaxial – many planes, sagittal, frontal, horizontal with corresponding axes.	Movements – flexion extension, adduction, abduction, rotation (limited), circumduction
■ Ball and socket joints	Hip and shoulder joints. Multiaxial – many planes, sagittal, frontal, horizontal with corresponding axes.	Movements – flexion, extension, adduction, abduction, rotation (medial and lateral), circumduction.

The range of movement at joints

The range and degree of movement at joints will vary from individual to individual and will depend on many factors. An understanding of these differences will enable the therapist to plan realistic objectives and avoid being over ambitious.

- The shape and contour of the articulating surfaces.
- The tension of the connective tissue components – the capsule and the ligaments supporting the joint.
- The tension of muscles and tendons around the joint.
- The approximation of soft tissue near the joint.

■ Ageing will affect joint range: children are more supple than young adults, and the young adults more supple than the elderly because tissues and ligaments etc tighten with age.

Because of the importance of joint movements when giving exercises, the basic structure and movements of each joint must be clearly understood. This knowledge enables the therapist to select appropriate exercises to maintain range and mobility and most importantly to give advice on the prevention of injury, ie, strains, sprains, dislocation and fractures.

The four ranges of movement are fully discussed in Chapter 6.

The major features of skeletal joints

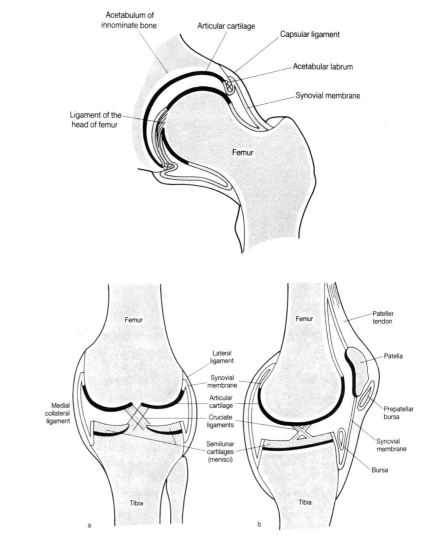

Figure 3.18 *A hip joint*

Figure 3.19 *A knee joint*
(a) viewed from the front
(b) viewed fron the side

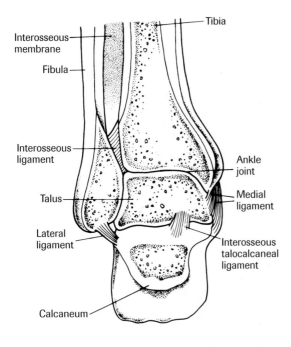

Figure 3.20   *An ankle joint*

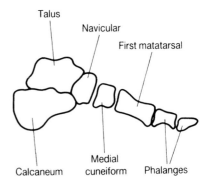

Figure 3.21   *The medial arch of the (left) foot*

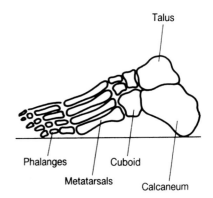

Figure 3.22   *The lateral arch of the (left) foot*

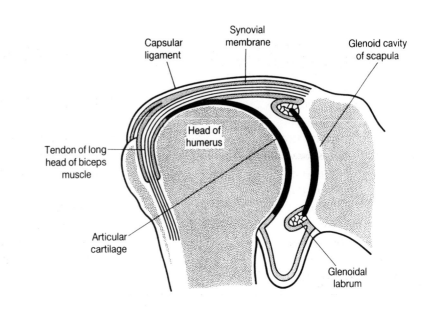

Figure 3.23   *The shoulder joint*

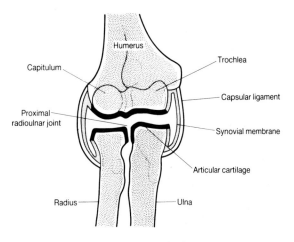

Figure 3.24   *The elbow joint*

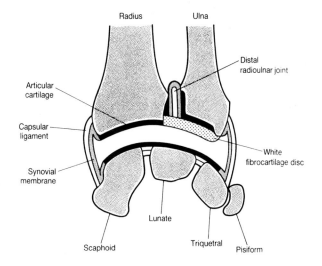

Figure 3.25   *The wrist joint*

Questions

1 Define the term *articulation*.
2 List the three main groups of joints and give an example from each group.
3 Give the functions of the following parts of a synovial joint:
   ▦ The synovial membrane;
   ▦ The synovial fluid;
   ▦ The hyaline cartilage.
4 Name one joint where discs or menisci are to be found.
5 List the six types of synovial joint.
6 Briefly explain any four factors which limit the range of movement at joints.
7 List and define the movements of the hip joint.
8 Give two reasons why there is a greater range of movement in the hip joint compared with the shoulder joint although both are ball and socket.
9 Give the movements of the ankle joint (remember that this is a hinge joint).
10 Name and describe the movements which occur between the radius and ulna.

Skeletal muscle

Muscles form the body flesh. Their function is to produce movement, maintain posture and produce body heat. Muscle tissue is totally under the control of the nervous system: impulses transmitted from the brain via motor nerves initiate contraction of muscle fibres. This contraction pulls on bones and movement occurs at joints.

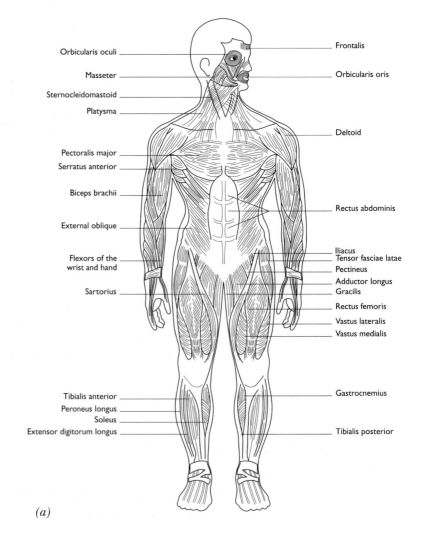

Figure 3.26   *The muscular system (a) anterior view (b) posterior view*   *(a)*

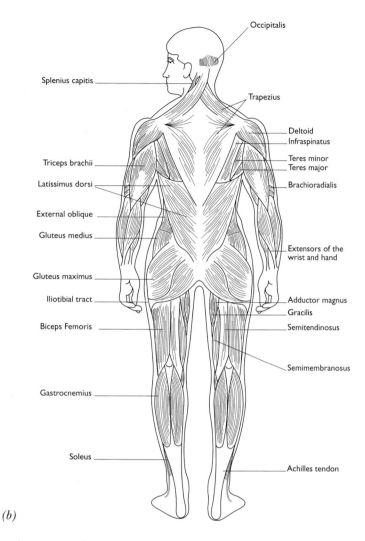

Occipitalis

Splenius capitis

Trapezius

Deltoid
Infraspinatus

Teres minor
Teres major

Triceps brachii

Brachioradialis

Latissimus dorsi

External oblique

Gluteus medius

Extensors of the
wrist and hand

Gluteus maximus

Iliotibial tract

Adductor magnus
Gracilis

Biceps Femoris

Semitendinosus

Semimembranosus

Gastrocnemius

Soleus

Achilles tendon

(b)

Structure of skeletal muscle

Skeletal muscle is composed of *muscle fibres* arranged in bundles called *fasiculi.* Many bundles of fibres make up the complete muscle. The fibres, bundles and muscles are surrounded and protected by connective tissue sheaths.

- The connective tissue around each fibre is called the *endomysium.*
- The connective tissue around each bundle is called the *perimysium.*
- The connective tissue around the muscle is called the *epimysium.*

This connective tissue blends at each end of the muscle to form tendons which attach the muscle to underlying bone.

Muscle fibres

Muscle fibres are long, thin, multinucleated cells. The fibres vary from 10–100 microns in diameter and from a few millimetres to many centimetres in length. The long fibres may extend the full length of the muscle, while the short fibres end in connective tissue intersections within the muscle.

Each muscle fibre is bound by a cell membrane known as the *sarcolemma* just beneath which lie the nuclei. The cytoplasm of the muscle cell is known as the *sarcoplasm*. It contains high numbers of mitochondria (where the enzymes for aerobic ATP are located) and other organelles. Muscle fibres are made up of smaller threads called *myofibrils*. These run the whole length of the fibre and are the elements which contract and relax.

Myofibrils are made up of even smaller threads called *myofilaments*. Under an electron microscope, myofibrils are

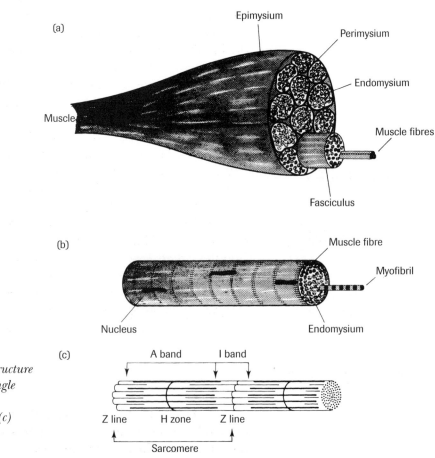

Figure 3.27 *(a) The structure of skeletal muscle (b) Single muscle fibre, showing characteristic striations (c) Myofibril, illustrating a sarcomere*

seen to have alternate light and dark bands called I and A bands. In the middle of the dark A band is a lighter zone, the H zone. In the middle of the light I band is a dark line, the Z line.

The segment between two Z lines is known as the *sarcomere*. These sarcomeres are repeated along the whole length of the myofibril. Each sarcomere contains overlapping thick and thin myofilaments. The thin myofilaments are made of the protein actin: they begin at the Z line and extend into the A band where they overlap with the thick myofilaments which are made of the protein myosin. These thick bands of myosin have small cross bridges projecting sideways towards active sites on the thin actin bands. These are very important and pull the thin actin bands towards the thick bands.

When a stimulus from the nervous system is received by the muscle fibre, a series of chemical reactions take place which results in the cross-bridges linking and pulling the thin bands into the thick bands. The sliding thin bands pull on the Z lines and each sarcomere shortens, consequently the myofibrils and fibres shorten and the whole muscle contracts. The energy for this contraction is obtained from the breakdown at ATP (*adenosine triphosphate*) stored in the myosine cross bridges.

Muscle relaxation occurs when no stimulus is received from the nervous system. The thin bands slide back to their precontracted state and the muscle relaxes. Muscle elongation only occurs as a result of some pulling force on the muscle. These forces may be the pull of antagonistic muscles (ie, on the opposite side of the joint), the pull of gravity, or the pull of weights, springs etc or the manual pulling by self or another person.

The fibres elongate because the thin filaments move away from the thick filaments and each sarcomere gets longer. The pull must allow at least one crossbridge to remain intact otherwise the sarcomere will rupture. Strong forces can cause small tears within a muscle because the cross bridges are no longer intact. During exercise and sports, excessive stress may result in muscle tears.

Myosin filaments   Actin filaments

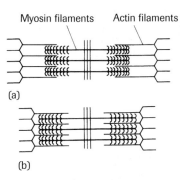

(a)

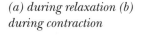

(b)

Figure 3.28   *The sarcomere (a) during relaxation (b) during contraction*

The all or none law

Stimuli from the brain and spinal cord are transmitted to a muscle fibre via its motor unit. When skeletal muscle fibres respond to nervous stimuli, the weakest stimulus which produces a contraction is known as the *threshold* stimulus. The threshold stimulus will produce a contraction of maximum force in the fibres supplied by the motor unit. Fibres do not respond with the partial contraction, ie, they contract with maximum force or not at all. This is known as the *all or none law*. However this is not true of the muscle as a whole. Muscle contraction may be weak or strong depending on the number of motor units stimulated. Different types of fibres within a muscle respond to stimuli of different frequencies, some will contract in response to a particular frequency while others will not. The strength of muscle contraction will also be affected by lack of nutrients, lack of oxygen or by the presence of lactic acid.

Muscle attachments

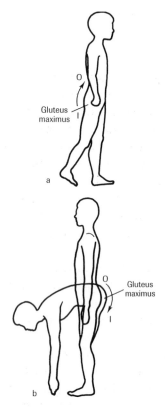

Gluteus maximus

Gluteus maximus

Figure 3.29   *Actions of the glueteus maximus (a) Extension of the hip joint, the insertion moves towards the origin (b) Raising the trunk, the origin moves towards the insertion*

As previously explained, a muscle is composed of muscle fibres and connective tissue components namely the endomysium, perimysium and epimysium. Certain muscles have connective tissue intersections dividing the muscle into several bellies as seen in the rectus abdominus.

These sheets of connective tissue blend at either end of the muscle and attach the muscle to underlying bones. Muscles are attached via *tendons* or *aponeuroses* to the periosteum covering the bone.

■ *Tendons* are tough cord-like structures of connective tissue which attach muscles to bones.
■ *Aponeuroses* are flat sheets of connective tissue which attach muscles along the length of bone.

A muscle has at least two points of attachment known as the *origin* and *insertion* of the muscle. These are attached on either side of a joint:

■ The *origin* is usually proximal and stationary or immovable.
■ The *insertion* is usually distal and movable.

When muscles contract, it is usual for the insertion to move towards the origin which remains stationary. However, certain muscles can also work in reverse, origin moving towards insertion. This is known as 'the reverse action of muscles' or 'origin insertion reversed'. For example, gluteus maximus extends the hip joint. When it pulls the leg backwards, the insertion on the femur moves towards the origin on the pelvis which remains stationary. However if the trunk is in forward flexion, gluteus maximum can pull the trunk upright when its origin on the pelvis moves towards the insertion on the femur which remains stationary. This is the reverse action.

Muscle shape

Muscle shape varies depending on the function of the muscle (see Figure 3.30, page 61). The fleshy bulk of the muscle is known as the belly. The muscle fibres forming bundles lie parallel or obliquely to the line of pull of the muscle. Parallel fibres are found in strap like and fusiform muscles. These long fibres allow for a wide range of movement. Oblique fibres are found in triangular and pennate muscles. These shorter fibres are found where muscle strength is required.

Blood supply to skeletal muscle

The circulating blood delivers supplies of oxygen and nutrients to the muscles and removes waste products such as carbon dioxide and lactic acid from the muscles. The arteries branch to form smaller arteries and arterioles within the perimysium and further divide, forming capillary networks within the endomysium. Here they join venules which lead to veins. When muscles are relaxed, the capillary networks deliver blood to the muscle fibres. When muscles contract, the pressure impedes the flow of blood through the capillary beds. This reduces the supply of oxygen and nutrients and limits removal of waste.

During exercise, muscle fibres alternately contract and relax and the capillaries deliver blood during the relaxation phase. However, if the contraction is sustained or prolonged as in isometric work or fast repetitive exercises, the blood vessels and capillaries are compressed. This impedes the free flow of blood to the muscle fibres, and limits the supply of oxygen and nutrients; waste products such as lactic acid accumulate which results in fatigue. The strength and speed of contraction becomes progressively weaker, as fatigue continues the muscle fails to relax completely, resulting in muscle spasm and pain.

Regardless of the activity, muscles must be given sufficient time to relax completely. This will ensure an adequate blood supply and prevent fatigue. Regular endurance aerobic exercise results in an increase in blood vessels and capillary networks to the muscles. This will improve the blood supply, increase levels of oxygen and nutrients and reduce levels of lactic acid. Thus the capacity to exercise without fatigue will improve.

Muscle tone

Muscle tone is the state of partial contraction or tension found in muscles even when at rest. A small number of muscle fibres will always be in a state of contraction. This is sufficient to produce tautness in the muscle, but not to result in full contraction and movement. Different groups of fibres contract alternately, working a 'shift' system to prevent fatigue of the few. Changes in muscle tone are adjusted according to the information received from sensory receptors within the muscles and their tendons. *Muscle spindles* transmit information on the degree of stretch within the muscle. *Tendon receptors* called Golgi organs transmit information on the amount of tension applied to the tendon by muscle contraction. Too much stretch and tension will be counteracted by a reduction in muscle tone. Too little will be counteracted by an increase in muscle tone. Muscle tone is essential for maintaining upright posture.

■ Hypotonic muscles, i.e. those with less than the normal degree of tone, are said to be flaccid.
■ Hypertonic muscles, i.e. those with a greater degree of muscle tone and where fibres are over-contracted and rigid, are said to be spastic.
■ A contraction that increases muscle tone but does not change the length of the muscle is called isometric contraction (equal tone).
■ A contraction where muscle tone remains the same but the muscle changes in length is called isotonic contraction (equal tone).

Energy for muscle contraction

All cells require energy for cellular activity. Muscle cells expend far more energy than other cells, and convert chemical energy to mechanical energy. Energy for muscle contraction is supplied by the high energy phosphate, adenosine triphosphate (ATP). The breakdown of ATP releases energy, which triggers the rowing action of the myosine cross bridges and hence the sliding action of muscle contraction. When muscles are at rest, ATP and phosphocreatine stores build up within the muscles, together with glycogen, triglycerides and enzymes. These enzymes act as catalysts to the energy generating chemical reactions that occur in muscle cells. (A catalyst is a chemical which changes the rate of a reaction but remains unchanged itself.)

- If the energy is generated by reactions which do not utilise oxygen, they are termed *anaerobic* energy systems.
- If the reactions utilise oxygen, they are termed *aerobic* energy systems.

The availability and use of oxygen is related to the intensity and duration of the exercise. Short bursts of intense activity require high energy production for a short time, but oxygen cannot be supplied fast enough. Steady state long duration activities require prolonged low energy production, which gives the body systems time to take in, deliver and utilise oxygen.

The anaerobic system

When a muscle is stimulated to contract, immediate energy is obtained from stored ATP; after 5–6 seconds of activity, the ATP is used up and must be replenished by the breakdown of phosphocreatine. This is known as the *phosphate* energy system or *alactic* system, and is anaerobic because oxygen is not utilised. Energy is supplied for 10–15 seconds, until the supply of phosphocreatine is depleted (it is therefore suitable for 100 metre sprints, or short intense actions such as pushing off the starting block or throwing actions). If the activity continues, more ATP must be manufactured from the breakdown of glycogen or fat.

If the activity is intense, the cardiovascular system is unable to provide oxygen fast enough to complete the breakdown of glycogen. ATP is resynthesised from the partial breakdown of glycogen to pyruvic acid and lactic acid, which accumulates in the blood and in the muscles. This is known as the *lactate* energy system (no oxygen is utilised, so it is also an anaerobic energy system). This system yields only two molecules of ATP per molecule of glucose, and so the body's glycogen stores are quickly depleted. This system will produce fast energy for up to 2–3 minutes, and will result in the build up of lactic acid and incur oxygen debt (see page 60). This will limit muscle contraction if the intensity of the activity is maintained, and exhaustion will result.

The aerobic system

Energy for prolonged medium to low intensity activity is generated through the complete breakdown of glycogen obtained from carbohydrates and fats to yield ATP, carbon dioxide and water. These reactions require oxygen and are therefore known as aerobic energy systems.

- Carbohydrates are the chief source of energy, and are stored as glycogen in muscle tissues and in the liver.
- Fats are the second source of energy, stored as fatty acids and triglycerols in muscle and adipose tissue.
- Protein is only used under extreme conditions of starvation or ultra marathon running.

The proportions of carbohydrates and fats used will depend on availability, and on the intensity and duration of the exercises. As intensity increases, a greater proportion of carbohydrates is used, but as duration increases, fats are utilised. The body stores far more fat than glycogen and so very rarely runs out of this fuel, but it can run out of glycogen. This will limit endurance activities because a small amount of glycogen must be available for fat to burn ('fat burns in a carbohydrate flame'). When marathon runners 'hit the wall', they are running out of glycogen; protein will be used when these sources become depleted.

This energy system is capable of producing far more energy than the anaerobic system. Each glucose molecule will yield 38 molecules of ATP. Providing a supply of oxygen can be maintained, muscle contraction can continue indefinitely until exhaustion is reached, as there is no lactic acid build up to cause muscle fatigue. If the intensity of the exercise should increase to such a degree that the cardiovascular system is unable to supply oxygen fast enough, then the anaerobic system will switch in.

The aerobic system is used in jogging, swimming,

running, cross-country skiing, cycling, aerobic dance and other aerobic exercises. The activity must be steady state and below maximal effort, to allow the systems to deliver and utilise oxygen.

Training for aerobic fitness will:

■ increase the intake of oxygen and transportation to the cells
■ increase the enzymes required to metabolise the glucose and fat
■ increase the use of fat as the energy source.

Fat needs a great deal of oxygen for its breakdown, therefore, by increasing oxygen uptake, fat will provide fuel. This spares the glycogen, it will last longer and the capacity to exercise is increased.

Table 3.4 Summary of anaerobic and aerobic systems

Anaerobic (Alactic) ATP-PC system	Anaerobic (Lactic Acid system)	Aerobic (Oxygen system)
Uses stored ATP and PC	Uses glycogen	Uses glycogen, fatty acids, proteins in emergency
Beginning of all activities and very fast short bursts – 15 seconds	Fast activity – up to 2 minutes	Slow steady activity indefinitely
For example: quick dash, 100 metre sprint, throw	For example: 400 meter run, fast lifts	For example: jogging, cycling, swimming
Contraction stops when ATP and PC used up	Contraction stops due to lactic acid build up and build up of oxygen debt	Contraction maintained indefinitely until glycogen is depleted and exhaustion is reached

Oxygen uptake

Oxygen uptake is the amount of oxygen consumed within a certain time, usually one minute. It is expressed as **VO_2**. The amount of oxygen consumed at rest is around 0.2–0.3 litres per minute, but this increases considerably during exercise to around 3–6 litres per minute. (*Maximum oxygen uptake* ('VO_2 max') is the peak rate of oxygen consumption during maximal activity.) It is the difference between the volume of oxygen inspired and the volume expired. VO$_2$ max is also known as an individual's *aerobic capacity*.

VO$_2$ max can be measured and used to assess a person's aerobic power or fitness. Training improves fitness, ventilation increases, the heart pumps out more blood which is delivered to and used by the muscles more efficiently. As fitness increases, the volume of oxygen consumed increases. Comparing VO$_2$ max values taken throughout a training programme, gives an indication of the improvement achieved. Trained athletes have a far higher VO$_2$ max than untrained individuals.

■ Regular training increases the capacity for oxygen uptake and the ability to exercise aerobically for longer periods.

Oxygen debt

This is the term used when oxygen supplies are depleted during vigorous muscular activity, and oxygen cannot be supplied fast enough to the muscle fibres (see above). After the exercise has stopped, extra oxygen is required to metabolise the small percentage of lactic acid remaining in the muscle, replenish ATP, phosphocreatine and glycogen; increased oxygen supplies are also required in the blood and lungs in order to restore the body systems to their normal state. The increase of lactic acid in the blood stimulates the respiratory system so that breathing increases in depth – the oxygen debt is then repaid. (Any lactic acid remaining in the muscles will inhibit their contraction.)

■ *Aerobic exercise* (endurance exercises which utilise oxygen for energy production): Oxygen supply is maintained throughout aerobic exercise, and a debt is not incurred. There is therefore no gasping or deep breathing at the end of these activities. If the exercises become too fast and vigorous, they will be anaerobic. Remember that clients should not be short of breath during aerobic activities and should be able to talk or sing while exercising.
■ *Anaerobic exercise* (activities which do not use oxygen for energy production): Oxygen debt is incurred during anaerobic exercise, which must be repaid at the end of the activity by deep breathing.

Muscle fatigue

Muscle fatigue is the inability of a muscle to sustain a contraction. The contraction becomes progressively weaker and then fails completely as the muscle is unable to produce sufficient energy to meet its needs. Muscle fatigue is thought to be due to depletion of ATP, insufficient glycogen and oxygen, and to the build up of lactic acid within a muscle.

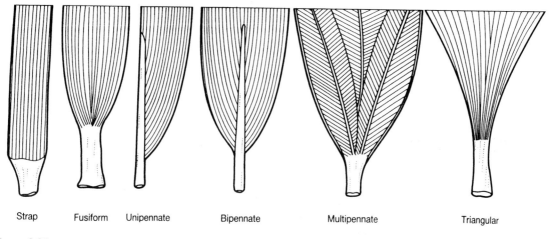

Strap   Fusiform   Unipennate   Bipennate   Multipennate   Triangular

Figure 3.30   *Muscle shape*

Questions

1 Give three functions of muscle tissue.
2 Name two contractile proteins found in muscle fibres.
3 Explain what happens to a muscle fibre if the cross bridges do not remain intact.
4 Discuss the 'All or None Law' related to muscle contraction.
5 Explain the following terms:
   ■ Tendon
   ■ Aponeurosis
   ■ Origin
   ■ Insertion.

6 Define the terms:
   ■ Hypotonic
   ■ Hypertonic.
7 Name the chemical compound which provides energy for muscle contraction.
8 Explain the terms:
   ■ anaerobic energy systems
   ■ aerobic energy systems.
9 Explain what is meant by the term 'VO$_2$ maximum'.
10 Define the term 'muscle fatigue' and explain how it may occur.

CHAPTER 4

Nutrition and Diet

This is a vast and specialised field, the detail of which is not within the scope of this book. Therapists requiring detailed information should therefore refer to specialist texts. However, this chapter should provide you with a solid foundation for this important topic.

The food we eat is broken down by the digestive system and used to maintain body functions such as

- providing energy for cellular activity
- providing building material for tissue growth and repair
- producing hormones, enzymes and antibodies.

A good balanced diet must be eaten to supply all the nutrients necessary for the body to perform its functions and promote health. Any food which is surplus to requirements is converted into fat and stored in adipose tissue. These fat stores are our fuel storage tanks; in times of high demand or low calorie intake, this fat is removed and broken down to provide energy for muscle contraction.

Energy

Energy may be defined as the capacity to perform work. The energy requirements of the body will vary depending on the activities carried out. The basic energy requirement of the body for maintaining body functions in the waking state, is known as the *basal metabolic rate* (BMR). This refers to the condition of the body first thing in the morning before getting up, or after lying down for at least 60 minutes. BMR is proportional to body weight: the heavier you are, the higher your BMR will be. It is generally higher for men and decreases with age. The demand for energy will proportionally increase as body activities increase; ie, the greater the intensity of the activity, the greater the energy expenditure will be.

Calories

A calorie is a unit of heat used to express the energy value of food.

- A calorie is the heat required to raise the temperature of one gram of water by 1 degree Celsius.
- A Kilocalorie (Kcal) is the heat required to raise one Kilogram of water by 1 degree Celsius.

The metric measurement of the energy value of food is the kilojoule. To convert Kcal to KJ:

1 Kcal = 4.2 KJ

Calorie intake should never be below one's basal metabolic rate; low calorie diets of 1,000 Kcals or below are dangerous. A well balanced diet of around 1,500 Kcals per day should provide adequate nutrients for those leading sedentary lives, but most people require more. The average active female consumes over 2,000 Kcals per day and the average male consumes over 3,000 Kcals. However, for anyone involved in intense physical activity, eg, athletes, sports people etc., this will rise to 4,000–6,000 Kcals and above. These individuals must carefully consider their diet to ensure that they are meeting their energy demands.

Essential nutrients

There are 6 basic nutrients necessary for a healthy diet:

- carbohydrates
- fats (lipids)
- proteins
- vitamins
- minerals
- water.

Fibre is an additional requirement, as it aids the functioning of the digestive tract and protects against many diseases.

Carbohydrates, fats and proteins are the energy providers and are known as *energy nutrients* or *macronutrients*. The other nutrients play important roles but they do not provide energy; they are known as *micronutrients*. Other chemical compounds derived from plants known as *phyto chemicals* have recently been identified which offer protection against carcinogens (substances which produce cancer).

Carbohydrates

Carbohydrates give the body its source of quick energy, and are the starches, sugars and cellulose found in pulses, cereals, bread, honey, potatoes, pasta, rice, and root vegetables. They are composed of carbon, hydrogen, and oxygen.

Carbohydrates are divided into three main groups:

1 Monosaccharides (glucose, fructose and galactose)
2 Dissaccharides (sucrose, lactose and maltose)
3 Polysaccharides (starches, glycogen, and cellulose).

During digestion, complex sugars (polysaccharides) are broken down to simple sugars (disaccharides) and then to one unit sugars (monosaccharides). These are absorbed in the small intestine and transported in the blood to the liver, where fructose and galactose are converted to glucose.

Sources of carbohydrate in our diet

Simple carbohydrates (monosaccharides and disaccharides) are the sugars found in honey, syrups, jams or fruits etc. They give a quick surge of energy which quickly disappears, making us feel tired and craving for more. Sugar and refined carbohydrates (white flour, white rice etc.) are low in vitamins, minerals and fibre and are therefore not as nutritious as unrefined and complex carbohydrates.

Complex carbohydrates (polysaccharides) are starches and fibre. They are found in bread, cakes, pasta, cereals, pulses, fruit and vegetables. They should form the greater percentage of our dietary intake because they provide vitamins, minerals, fibre and phyto chemicals. *Unrefined,* wholemeal products (eg, brown rice, wholemeal bread and pasta) have a high nutritional value.

Glucose

Glucose obtained from the breakdown of carbohydrates is used to produce ATP (adenosine triphosphate) required for muscle contraction (see p. 56). After eating a meal, blood sugar (glucose) levels will rise, which stimulates the pancreas to secrete insulin. Insulin reduces blood sugar levels, as it aids the transport of glucose from the blood into the cells. Glucose is then either used directly by the cells for immediate energy, or is converted in the liver to glycogen by a process known as *glycogenesis*. This glycogen is then stored in the liver or in muscle tissue, and will provide a reserve of energy for future use. When these stores are full, surplus glucose is converted in the liver to fat, which is then stored as triglycerides in adipose tissue. Thus, a low fat but high carbohydrate diet may still increase body fat if all the carbohydrate is not utilised for energy.

When energy demands are high, stored glycogen is needed. The liver then converts glycogen back to glucose, to supply the energy required. This process is known as *glycogenolysis*.

■ One gram of carbohydrate yields approximately 4.0 Kcals of energy

The body is only able to store a small amount of glycogen – around 500 g – which amounts to around 2000 Kcals of energy. Of this, approximately 80% is stored in skeletal muscle tissue and 20% in the liver. This is only enough to provide energy for one day of normal activity, so a regular intake of carbohydrate is necessary to maintain glycogen stores.

The average person with a sedentary life style should derive over 50% of total daily calories from carbohydrates (this means consuming over 300 g daily). The athlete or anyone with high energy expenditure will require over 60–70% which means over 400–600 g daily.

The use of carbohydrates during exercise

Glycogen will be used to produce ATP during all forms of exercise, but the proportion used increases with the intensity and decreases with the duration of the activity. During short bursts of intense anaerobic activity, such as fast short duration sprints, stored ATP, phosphocreatine and glycogen provide the energy. During prolonged moderate or intense aerobic activity, carbohydrates will be the main source, but a proportion will be supplied by fats. Prolonged low intensity activity such as distance walking or jogging will use a greater percentage of fat.

Following any intense activity, muscle and liver glycogen will be depleted. It is important to restore glycogen levels as quickly as possible after exercise, by eating a high carbohydrate meal. The more depleted the store, the longer it will take to restore and the more carbohydrate will be required. It is recommended that 1 g of carbohydrate is eaten for every kilogram of body weight.

Exercising with low glycogen levels will lead to early muscle fatigue and poor performance. It is therefore vital for athletes, sports people etc. to ensure a high carbohydrate intake as this will enable them to exercise for longer and to improve performance.

Research has shown that a high carbohydrate diet significantly increases endurance. Long distance runners increase carbohydrate intake to around 80% of total calorie intake to enhance performance. These athletes may practise the technique of *carbohydrate loading*, to substantially increase glycogen stores. This involves depleting glycogen stores for three days through exercise and diet, followed by a high consumption of carbohydrates two to three days before the event. However, this is no longer recommended, and at most should only be done twice or three times a year, as it can lead to fatigue and health risks. Different techniques of carbohydrate loading are being introduced, including gradually decreasing the duration of training and increasing carbohydrate intake for seven days before performance.

During any activity of 60 minutes or over, carbohydrate intake can help to delay fatigue. Suitable consumables include carbohydrate sports drinks, or a banana.

Fats

Fats are the body's secondary source of energy: carbohydrates provide primary fast energy, while fats provide long-term energy. Like carbohydrates, they are composed of carbon, hydrogen, and oxygen but in a different ratio – there is less oxygen in fats. Fats or lipids are obtained from animal and vegetable sources.

Sources of fat in our diet

There are two main types of fat:

- saturated
- unsaturated.

Saturated fats

These contain the maximum number of hydrogen atoms in each molecule, and so are *saturated* with respect to hydrogen. They tend to be solid at room temperature. Saturated fats are found mainly in animal products such as pork, beef, lamb, butter, milk, cheese, eggs etc. They are also found in certain plant products such as cocoa butter, palm oil and coconut oil. These fats contribute to high blood cholesterol levels and heart disease, and their excessive consumption should be discouraged.

Unsaturated fats

These contain fewer hydrogen atoms, and so are called *unsaturated*. This group include monounsaturated fats and polyunsaturated fats. These come mainly from plant sources, and tend to be liquid at room temperature.

- Monounsaturates include olive oil and peanut oil.
- Polyunsaturates include corn oil, sunflower oil, sesame oil, cotton seed oil, soybean oil.

These fats help to reduce cholesterol levels; the consumption of these fats, in particular the monosaturates, is preferable to saturated fats.

The use of fats during exercise

Both saturated and unsaturated fats provide the same amount of energy per unit weight:

- One gram of fat yields approximately 9.0 Kcals of energy

In addition to providing energy, fats protect vital organs such as the heart and kidneys, they provide body insulation, and are used in many physiological processes such as resynthesising tissues; eg, the myelin sheaths of nerves and thromboplastin for blood clotting. They also transport the fat soluble vitamins.

During digestion, fats are broken down to fatty acids and glycerol. If these fatty acids are not required for immediate energy, they are converted and stored in adipose tissue and in the liver in the form of triglycerides.

Fats are the body's most concentrated source of energy. Twice as much energy is stored in one gram of fat, than in one gram of carbohydrate. The body is able to store far more fat than glycogen, and so a greater store of potential energy which allows us to exercise for very long periods; even marathon runners do not run out of fat. However, fat requires a small amount of glycogen for its combustion and if glycogen stores are depleted, fat cannot be broken down to provide energy.

Fat cannot provide energy for fast activity, because it depends on the availability of oxygen, which depends on a person's aerobic capacity. A fit person with high aerobic capacity will burn fat more easily than an unfit person. During medium pace activities, fat provides around 50% of the required energy. If the effort is prolonged, fat will provide up to 90% of the required energy.

High fat intake increases the likelihood of developing high cholesterol levels, hypertension and heart diseases. It is also linked with the development of many cancers, such as breast and colon cancers. It is recommended that fat intake should not exceed 20–30% of total energy intake; of this, only 6–10% should be saturated fat.

Cholesterol

Cholesterol is a fatty like substance belonging to the chemical group known as *sterols*. Cholesterol is consumed in the diet, but is also synthesised in the liver. A high intake of saturated fat increases cholesterol levels, but it is also found in red meats, liver, kidney, egg yolk and dairy products. (It is not found in vegetables.) A certain amount of cholesterol is needed by the body for building cells and producing hormones, but too much is harmful, as it contributes to plaque formation in the arteries, which causes blockages and clots and increases the risk of coronary heart disease.

Cholesterol is bound to two types of lipoproteins:

1 high density lipoproteins (HDL) – this is 'good' cholesterol as it does not adhere to vessel walls and may even protect against heart disease.
2 low density lipoproteins (LDL) – this is the 'bad' high risk cholesterol.

A low intake of saturated fats and cholesterol rich foods is recommended to protect against heart disease.

Proteins

Proteins are chemically different from carbohydrates and fats, and are more complex in structure. They are composed of carbon, hydrogen and oxygen, but also contain nitrogen, sulphur and iron.

Proteins are the tissue builders of the body, used for growth, body building and tissue repair. Proteins are:

- used in the growth and repair of keratin, collagen, elastin
- used in the production of actin and myosin, which increase the size of myofibrils and the strength of muscle contraction
- needed to repair damage following injuries such as bone fractures, muscle strains, tendon and ligamentous injuries etc.
- essential in rebuilding muscle cells after intense effort
- catalysts for many chemical reactions
- thought to have an effect on the nervous system, increasing arousal and alertness, which are important for the elite performer
- used for making antibodies, enzymes and hormones.

Proteins are constructed from amino acids. There are 20 amino acids required by the body, and most can be manufactured by the body. However, eight cannot, and must be taken in from the diet; and these are known as *essential amino acids.*

Proteins are manufactured in the cells of plants and animals. Those containing all the essential amino acids are called *complete proteins* (high quality proteins). These are generally obtained from animal sources such as lean meat, fish, eggs, milk and cheese. Those which do not contain all the essential amino acids are called *incomplete proteins* (low quality), which are obtained from plant sources such as grains, pulses, fruit and vegetables. Vegans and vegetarians must ensure that they eat a wide variety of these products, to ensure an adequate intake of essential amino acids.

Food containing protein is broken down by the digestive system into amino acids. Those taken directly into cells are synthesised into new proteins, and the remainder are taken to the liver where some are synthesised into plasma proteins, others are de-animated and used for energy if required, or converted to glycogen or fat and stored.

There are no protein stores in the body, unlike carbohydrate and fat stores. All body protein is functional, therefore the body must ingest enough protein to meet its needs. Protein intake should be 10–15% of total energy intake; ie, 70–100 g per day (or 1 g for every kilogram of body weight). This should increase in times of illness, growth, tissue repair, during pregnancy or training and performance. Many elite performers increase their protein intake with supplements of amino acids (but there is no evidence to date to prove that taking supplements enhances performance).

■ One gram of protein yields 4.0 Kcals of energy

Proteins are only used as an energy source in cases of starvation, or very long distance running when all stores of carbohydrates and fats are running low.

Vitamins

Vitamins are chemical compounds. They are essential nutrients which enable the body to function efficiently, but they do not provide energy. They do however play important roles:

■ they regulate metabolic processes
■ they are important for growth, for the functioning of the nervous system and the immune system
■ they are involved in enzyme production, and in many other biological functions.

Vitamins are obtained from plant and animal food sources, and a balanced diet will ensure an adequate intake. Vitamins K and B_6 are formed by bacterial action in the large intestine, but the others must be obtained from the diet.
Vitamins may be grouped into:

■ Fat soluble vitamins (A, D, E, K)
■ Water soluble vitamins (B complex and C)

Fat soluble vitamins are stored in the liver and in fatty tissue whereas water soluble vitamins are excreted in the urine.

Fat soluble vitamins

Vitamin A

Source: fish oils, butter, milk, cheese, eggs. Our body can produce this vitamin from *carotenoids*; eg, beta-carotene found in yellow vegetables and fruits such as carrots, peaches, apricots, melon and in green leafy vegetables such as spinach and broccoli.
Function: aids growth and repair of tissues; maintains

mucous membranes, epithelial linings, and skin. Provides a visual pigment required for night vision. Beta-carotene may protect against heart attack, cancer, and reduce muscle soreness.
Deficiency: nightblindness.

Vitamin D

Source: fish oils, eggs, dairy products, fortified cereals, margarines. Produced in the skin by the action of sunlight on dehydrocholesterol.
Function: increases the absorption of calcium; promotes the growth of bones.
Deficiency: rickets, brittle bones and bone deformities.

Vitamin E

Source: Wheatgerm, wholemeal cereals and bread, nuts, seeds, egg yolk, vegetable oils.
Function: As an antioxidant it helps to protect against cancer, heart disease; it protects cell membranes; it helps muscles to utilise oxygen and may aid recovery after exercise.
Deficiency: possibly anaemia.

Vitamin K

Source: green vegetables, fruits, cereals, meat.
Function: involved in the formation or prothrombin; essential in blood clotting.
Deficiency: increased risk of haemorrhages.

Water soluble vitamins

Vitamin B complex

This is a large group of vitamins; each has a particular function.
Source: obtained from a wide variety of sources: lean meats, vegetables, pulses, legumes, whole grains, dairy products, eggs.
Function: They are essential for

- creating energy
- converting carbohydrates into glucose
- the metabolism of fats and proteins.

Some are associated with the manufacture of red blood cells, the growth and development of cells, and with the functioning of the nervous system.

Deficiency: as this group of vitamins has a wide range of functions, deficiency will result in many disorders and conditions – beriberi, pellagra, fatigue, muscular twitching, anaemia, nervous disorders, gastrointestinal problems.

Folic acid: this is included in the B vitamins. It helps to form heme, the iron containing protein which is needed to form red blood cells. It protects coronary vessels and is required for brain development and function.

Vitamin C

Source: citrus fruits, berries, tomatoes, peppers, leafy green vegetables.

Function: growth and tissue repair; collagen formation; important for healthy gums, teeth and blood vessels; it helps to absorb iron and utilise folic acid; it forms adrenaline; it helps fight bacteria, is an antioxidant and may help fight cancer.

Deficiency: scurvy, anaemia, poor connective tissue growth and repair, tender swollen gums and loose teeth, bleeding, decrease in exercise performance as it affects aerobic capacity.

Minerals

Minerals are found in all body cells and fluids, and they form part of the body's structure. Although these elements are only required in small quantities, they are essential for regulating and maintaining life processes. They cannot be manufactured by the body and must be obtained from the diet.

Calcium

Calcium is required for the formation of teeth and bones. Inadequate intake of calcium results in porous bones, known as *osteoporosis*. Menopausal women are particularly susceptible to this disease, as there is a loss of bone mass and a high risk of sustaining bone fractures. Regular exercise, an active lifestyle and an adequate calcium intake will protect against this disease.

Iron

Iron is an important mineral, as it is a component of haemoglobin and muscle myoglobin. An adequate iron intake is therefore important for transportation and the storage of oxygen. Female athletes in particular must guard against iron deficiency (anaemia), as this will affect aerobic capacity.

Other minerals such as **sodium**, **potassium** and **magnesium** are important for nerve impulse conduction and fluid balance. **Iodine** is required for proper functioning of the thyroid gland.

Profuse sweating will result in water and mineral loss which must be replaced through a balanced diet. Sports drinks can help in cases of severe fluid loss.

Vitamin and mineral requirements of the athlete

Manufacturers imply that the athlete will derive great benefit from taking vitamin and mineral supplements. These micronutrients do *not* provide energy, and research indicates that there is no benefit in consuming extra vitamins if recommended levels are maintained through a varied and balanced diet. It is true that these nutrients are essential for the proper functioning of bodily processes but they are only required in small amounts.

Nutritional requirements will vary depending on age, size, levels of activity and metabolism. Individuals who are very active will require more than those who are inactive, but because they generally eat more, they will obtain an adequate supply of nutrients naturally from food. Supplements may be advisable for those who are restricting calories or for vegans; they may also be recommended following illness, during pregnancy, or for those suffering from anaemia or other deficiency diseases.

Performance may be adversely affected if the intake of vitamins and minerals is below the recommended levels, but providing intake meets the recommended levels, performance will not be further improved by consuming large doses above this level. Advice should be sought from a doctor or qualified nutritionist before taking supplements.

When deficiency has been investigated and established, supplements must be limited to the recommended dose, and balanced to include all the nutrients which contribute in some way to performance. For example:

- vitamin A, for repair of tissues
- vitamin B complex, involved in energy metabolism
- vitamin C, necessary for the absorption of iron and the forming of red blood cells which transport oxygen
- vitamins C, E and beta-carotene to neutralise free-radicals, thus limiting post exercise pain and soreness (explained below)
- calcium, for strong bones
- iron, to improve the oxygen capacity of the blood
- magnesium, for nerve-muscle function, regulation of body temperature and to activate the enzymes involved in energy production
- potassium and sodium, for nerve-muscle function
- phosphorus as part of ATP, for energy release
- zinc, for tissue growth and repair and as a part of the enzymes required for metabolism of macro-nutrients.

Chemicals which affect the body

Free radicals

Free radicals are reactive chemicals; they are unstable atoms or molecules with unpaired electrons. They are continually produced in the body as a result of metabolic reactions, and are constantly trying to pair up with other electrons to regain stability. In their effort to become stable, they bombard other cells, damaging the cells and their DNA.

They may damage skin cells causing ageing, liver spots or skin cancers; they also damage the cells of other tissues producing various types of cancer. They attack and oxidise LDL cholesterol in the blood stream, resulting in a 'furry' plaque which blocks arteries and increases the risk of heart disease. Research has shown that there is a marked rise in free radical levels following exercise, and that they may be responsible for post exercise pain and stiffness. Fortunately substances have been identified that counter the effects of free radicals, which are known as **antioxidants**.

Antioxidants

These act as scavengers, neutralising free radicals and thus protecting the body from damage. Some are found in the body as parts of enzymes, whereas others must be consumed in the diet; eg, vitamins C, E and beta carotene, minerals such as zinc, copper, selenium and the many phyto chemicals found in fruit and vegetables. Research indicates that these phyto chemicals afford effective protection against free radicals and cancer.

Phyto chemicals

These are chemicals such as flavonoids, sulphoraphane and chlorogenic acid. They are found in fruits and plants, which, when eaten in adequate amounts, protect the body from carcinogens and promote health.

Research indicates that at least five portions of fruit and vegetables should be eaten daily. The following fruits and vegetables will provide a variety of different phyto chemical, each having different protective effects:

- Broccoli, cauliflower, cabbage, sprouts, kale, tomatoes, peppers, pineapples, strawberries, grapes, raspberries, onion, garlic and soya beans.

In fact, most fruit and vegetables offer some form of protection.

Water and other liquids

Water represents 40–70% of total body mass. Individuals who are lean and muscular have a higher water content than fatter individuals with the same body mass, because fat contains less water. The body does not store water – it is excreted in urine. If water loss is high, the body will quickly become **dehydrated** and death will occur within days. Under normal conditions, the body maintains a balance between fluid intake and output; feelings of thirst indicate that the body is dehydrated and that water is needed.

Water is essential for the biological functioning of the body:

- it plays a vital role in regulating body temperature
- substances dissolve in water and are transported around the body in blood plasma and lymph
- it is a component of cells and tissue fluid and provides a medium for the exchange of oxygen, nutrients and waste products between cells and the blood
- as part of synovial fluid, it lubricates joints and reduces friction
- it bathes tissues such as the eyes, brain and spinal cord
- waste products are excreted in water, as urine and faeces
- it absorbs heat and cools the body through evaporation. Dehydration occurs quickly during vigorous activity through profuse sweating and expired air.

To maintain water balance, the average person with a sedentary lifestyle should drink between two and three litres of water or diluted fruit juices every day. This is in addition to any tea, coffee or alcohol consumed because these are diuretics, which increase fluid loss.

Although it is a very unusual occurrence, it is important to remember that drinking *too* much water (over nine to ten litres per day) is dangerous. This will produce symptoms such as headache, blurred vision, sweating and vomiting. In extreme cases the brain is affected and the person becomes delirious, comatosed and may eventually die.

Dehydration during exercise

Contracting muscles generate a great deal of heat during exercise, up to 100 times more than resting muscles. The body must get rid of this extra heat, or the core body temperature will rise to dangerous levels. The blood transports this heat from the muscles to the skin surface where it is lost through convection, radiation and evaporation (sweating). In hot weather, there is little or no heat loss through convection and radiation, therefore heat loss must be through evaporation with increased sweating.

Vigorous activity produces profuse sweating, which can result in a fluid loss of 4–5% of body mass. The longer and harder the exercise and the hotter and more humid the conditions, the greater the fluid loss. Long distance runners may lose as much as two litres every hour through the lungs and skin. As fluid loss increases, the body becomes dehydrated. Water will be lost from all body compartments and there will be a reduction in blood volume. Because there is less blood for the heart to pump per beat, cardiac output is reduced, which in turn reduces the delivery of oxygen and nutrients to the contracting muscles; performance will be limited. The circulatory system tries to maintain blood volume to the muscles by constricting vessels and reducing blood flow to the skin, therefore less heat is lost and temperature rises.

The symptoms of dehydration include: a decrease in level of performance, nausea, irritability, dizziness, fatigue, confusion and eventually complete exhaustion and collapse.

It is possible to prevent dehydration by ensuring an adequate intake of fluid before, during and after vigorous or prolonged activity. Performers are recommended to:

1 Drink plenty of water the day before the event.
2 Drink two cups of water two hours before the event.
3 Drink one cup of water about 15–30 minutes before the event.
4 Drink a quarter to half a cup every 15–20 minutes during the event (this is not necessary for events lasting up to 30 minutes).
5 Rehydrate fully after the event (this will depend on the degree of dehydration).

Recording the weight before and after performance will give an indication of how much water has been lost and how much needs replacing after exercise. For every 1 kilogram of weight lost, 1 litre of water should be drunk to restore balance.

Sports drinks

Drinking water alone may not be enough to rehydrate the body, as the electrolytic balance must also be considered. Drinking water quickly removes the feeling of thirst (to protect against low plasma electrolyte levels), and stimulates the kidneys to excrete urine. This occurs before rehydration is complete. It is important to continue drinking even if feelings of thirst have diminished. Sports drinks are continually being developed, containing sodium and/or carbohydrate (glucose) and other electrolytes. Many of these drinks contain a glucose polymer, which is an easily digestible form of complex carbohydrate. The main aim of these drinks is to speed up rehydration; those containing carbohydrate also maintain blood sugar levels, delay depletion of muscle glycogen, and thus increase endurance.

Research indicates that for athletes exercising at low intensity for up to an hour, water is as effective as expensive sports drinks for preventing dehydration. Exercising for this length of time will not utilise the glucose provided by sports drinks, and the sodium lost is easily replaced through diet.

However, when exercising for long duration at moderate to high intensity, sports drinks are recommended as they rehydrate faster, and if consumed during exercise, can enhance performance. The intake of glucose raises blood sugar levels and spares muscle glycogen, so that the muscles contract harder for longer. Sodium helps to retain water in the blood without inhibiting thirst; it also limits urine production, therefore hydration is faster.

Many nutritionists believe that the diets of most people are already too high in sodium and so do not require it as an addition to drinks. It must also be remembered that carbohydrates supply calories, and those athletes wishing to control weight should avoid the extra calories found in these drinks.

Sports drinks come in different concentrations and selection is important. There are three kinds of sports drinks:

1 hypotonic
2 isotonic
3 hypertonic.

Although all these drinks will rehydrate the body, the main difference lies in their rate of absorption which is dependent on their **osmolarity** (this refers to the concentration of solutes in a solution). A drink with low osmolarity will have fewer particles in solution than a drink with high osmolarity.

Hypotonic drinks

Hypo means: *less* than. These drinks have *low* osmolarity; they have a lower concentration of solutes (less particles), usually less than 4 grams of sugar per 100 ml. They pass quickly out of the stomach and are absorbed for fast rehydration. These are geared to the low/moderate, short duration (up to one hour) athlete. Water would be just as suitable under these conditions, but some will enjoy the flavour of these drinks and consequently drink more.

Isotonic drinks

Iso means: the *same*. These drinks have a higher concentration of solutes than hypotonic drinks and are absorbed at about the same rate as water. They contain 4–8 grams of sugar per 100 ml and will refuel and rehydrate. These drinks are geared to the endurance athlete, exercising for one to three hours; if consumed during performance, they provide extra glycogen.

Hypertonic drinks

Hyper means: *more* than. These drinks have a much higher osmolarity, and are more concentrated than isotonic drinks. They slow gastric emptying, and are absorbed more slowly than water. Contain over 8 grams of sugar per 100 ml, they rehydrate slowly, spare muscle glycogen and prolong endurance. These drinks are geared to the ultramarathon runners, cyclists and others who must maintain effort all day.

Fibre

Fibre provides roughage and bulk which stimulates peristalsis and facilitates the movement of waste through the large intestine for excretion. We obtain fibre from wholemeal foods (brown bread, rice and pasta) and from fruit and vegetables. An intake of 20–35 grams per day is recommended. High fibre intake:

- reduces the risk of heart disease
- helps to lower cholesterol level
- decreases the risk of cancer, particularly colon cancer
- reduces the risk of gastrointestinal problems and diseases
- protects against diabetes.

A high fibre diet must be accompanied by high fluid intake to keep the colon functioning efficiently.

Weight control

Weight control is largely a balance between energy input (food eaten) with energy output (energy used).

- If energy input equals energy output, weight remains stable (neither gained or lost).
- If energy input is greater than energy output, weight increases as the excess fuel is stored on the body as fat.
- If the energy input is less than energy output, weight is lost as fuel is taken from the fat stores.

Therefore the most effective way to lose weight is to eat less and increase the level of aerobic activity. Aerobic exercise is the most effective form of activity for losing weight, as it utilises fat as well as carbohydrate for energy.

Any diet should aim at reducing weight by around 1 kilo per week. It is important to eat a balanced and varied diet and to include each of the foods necessary for health. It is potentially dangerous to reduce calorie intake to 1,000 cals or under. Most people will lose weight on a 1,500–2,000 cals diet. It is worth noting that:

- 1 gram of carbohydrate provides: 4 Kcals (17 kilojoules) of energy.
- 1 gram of protein provides: 4 Kcals (17 kilojoules) of energy.

but

- 1 gram of fat provides: 9 Kcals (39 kilojoules) of energy.

Therefore, eating more carbohydrate and protein and cutting down on fat will result in less energy intake and quicker weight loss.

Body composition

Body weight is dependent on the major structural components of the body, which include bone, muscle and fat. Weighing machines tell us how heavy we are, and by regularly weighing ourselves, we know whether we have gained or lost weight. We can also compare our weight against the so called 'norm' for our height, by checking established height–weight tables. If our weight is greater than the average values, we are classed as overweight; if our weight is less than the stated values, we are underweight. Being very overweight or very underweight can increase health risks. However it is important to remember that these are only 'average' values; we may not fit into the 'average mould', and weight alone tells us little about our individual state of health.

The **Body Mass Index** (**BMI**) is used to assess health risks in relation to weight and height. The BMI is calculated by dividing weight in kilograms, by the square of the height in metres. The result is then checked against the following risk table.

Table 4.1   Ranges of Body Mass Index

BMI Males			Diagnosis	BMI Females		
Light frame		**Heavy frame**		**Light frame**		**Heavy frame**
20	–	25	Acceptable	19	–	24
26	–	30	Overweight	25	–	29
31	–	40	Obese	30	–	40
41+			Dangerously obese	41+		

However, body **composition** is the important factor (ie, the ratio of fat to lean tissue). Too much fat increases the risk of developing many serious diseases such as hypertension, heart disease, vascular problems, stroke, diabetes, gall bladder disease, arthritis and certain cancers.

It is possible to be classed as overweight, even though the percentage of body fat is low. Many athletes and sports people develop large muscles through specific training which will add considerably to their weight. This is desirable weight gain from their point of view, and does not constitute a health problem. They may be overweight when compared with average tables, but they will not be 'overfat', which is the critical issue.

Although diet is the major factor in gaining fat, activity levels play a crucial part, as do other factors such as hormonal influences, inherited characteristics and somatotypes. These factors make it more difficult for some individuals to control their weight:

1 *Endomorphs:* These are short, stocky, curvaceous and plump. For this group weight/fat gain is easy but weight loss is difficult.
2 *Ectomorphs:* These are long limbed, slim and slightly muscular. They do not easily gain weight.
3 *Mesomorphs:* These are muscular and stocky. They gain weight/fat slowly but increase muscle strength easily.

Individuals are predominantly of one type but may have aspects of another.

Summary

Athletes and sportspeople require a low fat to lean tissue ratio, because fat means surplus baggage to carry around. This is costly in terms of energy expenditure which limits endurance. Transporting excess fat will increase inertia, reduce speed and agility. The greater the weight, the greater the inertia and the greater the effort required to overcome it. Fat laid down in muscle tissue increases friction which impairs strength and function. Some athletes and dancers reduce calories to dangerous levels in pursuit of leanness as it is aesthetically desirable and enhances performance. However, athletes must balance training and diet, and consume extra calories to meet high energy and muscle building requirements, but guard against fat gain.

High carbohydrate, moderate protein, low fat intake is recommended, together with an adequate intake of vitamins, minerals, water and fibre.

Obesity or high fat ratio (ie, 20% over desirable weight) is a major health problem in Western society. The majority of the population is too fat and should change their diet and increase exercise levels. A combination of healthy eating and increased levels of aerobic activity is the key to success. Regular, moderate/low intensity aerobic exercise of 20–30 minutes duration 3–5 times per week combined with reduced calorie intake around 2,000 calories per day will result in fat loss, improved body shape, and an increase in lean tissue. It is an advantage to have a high proportion of muscle tissue as it has a high metabolic rate, therefore more calories are burnt.

Quick guide to healthy eating

- Reduce intake fat, particularly saturated fat. When cooking boil, steam or bake food; do not fry.
- Reduce intake of red meat as it has high fat content, replace with poultry. Cut off all visible fat from meat and remove the skin from poultry. Avoid eating prepared foods such as sausages, pate, pies, etc.
- Reduce sugar and salt intake.
- Eat plenty of fish, particularly oily fish such as mackerel, salmon, herring, trout.
- Eat plenty of fresh or frozen vegetables – at least five portions per day (but do not overcook).
- Eat plenty of fresh, frozen or dried fruit.

- Eat wholemeal foods such as bread, pasta, rice, cereals, pulses, beans.
- Eat a wide variety of foods.
- Cut down on alcohol.
- Eat plenty of fibre.
- Drink two to three litres of water or diluted fruit juices per day.
- Low fat, high carbohydrate and moderate protein is recommended. Remember that fat has twice the number of calories as carbohydrate and protein (weight for weight).

Questions

1 Define the following terms
   - basal metabolic rate
   - kilocalorie
   - macronutrients
   - micronutrients
2 List the six basic nutrients necessary for a healthy diet.
3 Explain the importance of including plenty of fibre in the diet.
4 Give six examples of foods which provide carbohydrates.
5 Name the two main types of carbohydrates and give examples of where each is found.
6 Explain why a high carbohydrate intake is vital for distance runners.
7 List the two main types of fat and give examples of where each is found.
8 Compare the energy yield of one gram of fat with one gram of carbohydrate and protein.
9 Explain why a fit person with a high aerobic capacity will burn fat more easily than an unfit person.

10 Explain what is meant by the term 'essential amino acids'.
11 Define the terms:
   - Complete proteins
   - Incomplete proteins.
12 Name the fat soluble vitamins.
13 List four functions of vitamins.
14 Name two important minerals and give their function.
15 Explain what is meant by 'free radicals'. Why are they undesirable in the body?
16 Give three examples of antioxidants and explain their importance in the diet.
17 Explain why water is an important component of the diet.
18 Explain why vigorous exercise may result in dehydration.
19 Give the symptoms of dehydration.
20 Explain the difference between hypotonic, isotonic and hypertonic sports drinks.

CHAPTER 5

Physical Principles Relating to Exercise

The science or study of body movement is known as *kinesiology*. Movement is normally produced by the force of muscles pulling on bones, which results in movement at joints. When the body moves, it is also continually affected by external forces such as gravity, wind, friction etc. These forces will affect not only the movement of the human body but also the movement of any objects or projectiles used in sporting activity. The study of these forces and their effects is a branch of science known as *biomechanics*. An understanding of some of these scientific principles is required in order to analyse athletic performance and devise effective training practices which will enable the athlete or sportsperson to maximise effort and achieve peak performance. An explanation of terms will help the therapist to understand mechanical principles and concepts.

Explanation of terminology

Mass and weight: mass refers to the *quantity of matter* in a body. This differs from weight, which is the *force due to the gravitational field*. The mass of a body is the same everywhere, as it does not change with the gravitational field. An object will have the same mass, whether it is on the earth or on the moon (where gravitational pull is weak), but its weight will diminish as it moves out of the gravitational field.

Weight = Mass × gravitational field strength

Direction is the line of movement of an object.

Magnitude means largeness or size.

Scalar quantity refers to any physical quantity that has magnitude but no direction, such as speed or mass.

Vector describes a physical quantity that has both direction and magnitude, such as acceleration or velocity (note the difference from scalar quantity, which has magnitude but no direction).

Force is a push or pull which alters the motion of a body. Force has direction and magnitude and is therefore a vector. The force (F) applied by a body is equal to the mass (m) of the body multiplied by its rate of acceleration (a); this is expressed as:

$$F = m \times a$$

Velocity is the amount of distance travelled in a given time. As the distance over which a constant force is applied increases, velocity will increase. Discus or shot putters adopt starting positions which allow the force to be applied over the longest distance to gain maximum final velocity (the greater the velocity, the greater the distance the object will travel).

$$\text{Velocity} = \frac{\text{distance travelled}}{\text{time taken}}$$

Acceleration is an increase in the rate of speed; ie, the change of velocity per second. An increase in velocity per second is *positive* acceleration, whereas a decrease in velocity per second is *negative* acceleration (deceleration). Acceleration is proportional to the force producing it, if the mass is constant. A runner can increase his acceleration by increasing the force he applies to the running surface.

$$\text{Acceleration} = \frac{\text{change of velocity}}{\text{time taken}}$$

Speed is the distance travelled per second. The greater the force applied, the faster an object will travel.

Impetus is the force with which a body moves. It is the product of force and time, so that increasing the force or the time for which it acts, will increase the velocity of the body. The follow-through action in sport ensures that maximum force is applied for as long a time as possible.

Inertia is the reluctance of a body to change its current state of motion. It is directly proportional to the mass – the greater the mass, the greater the inertia.

Momentum is the quantity of motion of a moving body; it is the impetus gained by movement. It is a product of mass multiplied by velocity: momentum increases if the mass increases or if the velocity increases. If two athletes are moving with the same velocity, the one of larger mass will possess the greater momentum. The greater the momentum of a body, the greater the inertia – if a body has great momentum, it will be difficult to stop or change its direction.

Momentum = mass × velocity

Forces and their application

A force can be described as a push or pull which changes the state of motion of a body. Any force acting on a body will cause it to move or affect its movement. If a body is at rest, a force applied to it will make it move, providing the force is of sufficient magnitude to overcome the inertia of the body. If a body is already moving, a force will speed up the movement, slow it down, change its direction or stop it. When a force is applied, the outcome will depend on:

- the magnitude of the force
- the direction in which it is applied
- the point at which it is applied.

These three factors determine the resultant effect of the application of forces. Forces acting on the human body may be *internal* forces, eg, muscle contraction, or they may be *external* forces such as gravity, friction, weights, springs, pulleys, water etc.

Force is measured by the rate of change of momentum of the body on which it acts, ie, the mass of the body multiplied by its acceleration ($F = m \times a$).

It is measured in Newtons:

- 1 Newton is the force which makes a mass of 1 kilogram, accelerate by 1 metre per second squared.

When muscles contract, they exert a force which will produce movement at the underlying joint; eg, when we bend the elbow, the biceps muscle must contract with sufficient force to lift the forearm. The strength of the muscle must be great enough to overcome the resistance of any force pulling the other way, in this case the weight of the forearm. If an additional external force, such as a dumb bell in the hand, is applied, then the muscle force must be greater than the dumb bell and the weight of the forearm, for movement to occur. Muscles are strengthened when they are made to work against progressively increasing forces.

Certain postural muscles are continually working against

the force of gravity to maintain posture. If these muscles relaxed, the body would fall to the ground.

Types of forces

Forces may be applied singly, many forces may work together in the same direction or forces may work against each other (opposing forces). Below are examples of these forces in everyday life, muscle work and sport.

A single force

A single force acting on an object will move it in the direction of that force, if the force is great enough to overcome the mass of the object and its inertia. For example:

- A man pushing a car will move the car in the direction in which he is pushing, providing the force is great enough; the greater the force, the faster the car will move.
- A muscle pulling on a bone will move the bone, providing the muscle pull is strong enough. The stronger the muscle, the greater the force.
- A footballer kicking a ball will move the ball in the direction of the kick; the greater the force applied by his foot, the faster and further the ball will travel. The point at which he applies the force also affects the outcome. If he kicks the ball in the centre (ie, applies the force through the centre of gravity), the ball will travel in a straight line. If he strikes the ball off centre, the ball will curve and spin, and speed will be reduced (see page 89).

Two forces working together

If two or more forces are acting on the same point in the same direction, the magnitude of the force will be greater than either of the two forces. For example:

- Two men pushing a car at the same angle and in the same direction will move the car in the direction of the two forces. The magnitude of the force will be the force of the first man and the force of the second man, and the work will be easier for each man.

- In the same way, two muscles pulling together in the same direction will move a bone, and the work will be easier for each muscle than if they were working alone.
- A footballer kicking on a windy day will need to know the direction of the wind, as the wind provides another force. If he is kicking *with* the wind, he will need to exert less force than if there is no wind, to achieve the same distance.

Opposing forces

Two forces acting in opposite directions will result in movement in the direction of the greater force.

- Two men pushing a car in opposite directions will result in movement in the direction of the greater force.
- Opposing muscles cannot contract together because as the prime mover contracts, the opposing antagonist relaxes (this is controlled by nerve impulses and is known as *reciprocal relaxation*). However, muscles can be made to contract against external forces such as gravity, weights, springs, pulleys, machines. If the muscle force is greater than the external force, movement will occur in the direction of muscle pull. If the muscle force and the weight are equal, there will be no movement; ie, equilibrium will be reached. If the weight force is greater than the muscle force, movement will occur in the direction of the weight (if a muscle attempts to lift too great a weight, the myofibrils may tear, damaging the muscle).
- A footballer kicking a ball against the wind will need to overcome a greater resistance than if there was no wind, and will therefore need to apply a greater force to overcome that resistance.

Motion

A force is necessary to produce movement or motion. In sport and athletic performance, muscle contraction is the main force which produces the movements required. Movement or motion may be *linear* (translatory) or *angular* (rotary).

Linear motion

Linear motion takes place in a straight line (ie, movement from one point to another) and includes *curvilinear* motion when the pathway may curve. Linear motion is frequently followed by curvilinear motion due to the forces of resistance. For example: if a ball is thrown horizontally, its flight begins in a straight line, but it then curves downwards because of the force of gravity. Its flight may also be affected by other forces such as the wind direction and the point of application of the force.

A body which is freely movable will move in a straight line if a force is applied through its centre of gravity. If a ball is kicked and the force strikes through its centre of gravity, the ball will travel in a straight line. The distance and speed it travels will depend on the magnitude of the force and the opposing forces which resist its flight.

If a force is applied to a body at a point away from its centre of gravity, the body gains rotary motion which slows its linear motion.

Angular motion

Angular or rotary motion is movement around an axis or fulcrum when the axis lies within the mass; for example, twisting or spinning. Most activities in sport and athletics will be a combination of linear and angular motion. For example, a runner or swimmer will move forward with linear motion toward the line, due to the angular motion of the legs and arms. If, when a ball is kicked, the boot strikes away from the centre, the ball will spin and follow a curved path – its speed will be reduced if the magnitude of the force remains the same. The further away from the centre the force is applied, the faster the body will rotate.

The speed at which a body rotates will depend on its radius. When a skater performs a fast spin, the arms are drawn in close to the sides; to slow down the arms are extended, thus increasing the radius. The smaller the radius of movement, the faster the spin, if other factors are equal. This principle is used in diving: after the lift off the board, the diver tucks the body in, to gain more rotations.

Newton's Laws of Motion

The Laws of Motion devised by the scientist Sir Isaac Newton (1642–1727) explain the effects of forces. Any motion requires force to produce it, therefore some of the following principles have already been introduced.

Newton's three laws state:

1 A body will continue in a state of rest or uniform motion in a straight line unless it is acted on by a force (the law of **inertia**).
2 A change in acceleration of a body is directly proportional to the force, inversely proportional to the mass and takes place in the direction of the force (the law of **acceleration**).
3 To every action there is an equal and opposite reaction (the law of **counterforce**).

The first law – applied to sport

The first law refers to the resistance of a body to any change in motion. This applies not only to the human body, but also to any object. If a force is applied to a body at rest, it will make it move; if the body is moving, an applied force will change its speed, or the direction in which it is moving. As previously explained, if the force is applied in the same direction as the movement, the body will move faster; if the force is applied against the movement, the body will slow down. If the force applied against the movement is great enough, the object will stop. A force applied at an angle will change the direction of the movement. The greater the force applied, the greater will be the resultant change.

When performing an action, the athlete must produce considerable force and therefore expend a great deal of energy to overcome the body's resistance to movement (inertia). The larger and heavier the athlete, the greater will be the inertia and the more effort will be required to overcome it. Once movement is initiated, subsequent actions must follow smoothly without hesitation, or the advantage of overcoming inertia will be lost.

If the movement is linear, all the forces for increasing speed must be applied in that same direction for maximum effect. Forces applied in other directions will reduce the speed; eg, runners and swimmers must direct all possible forces forward and reduce any other forces to a minimum. With correct training practices, they learn to select and contract the appropriate muscles for applying these forward forces, and to cut out any inappropriate movements which waste energy and retard performance. Skilled performers maximise all appropriate forces and minimise extraneous movements.

The second law – applied to sport

This is the law of acceleration: the change in velocity of a body is directly proportional to the force acting on it and will take place in the direction in which the force acts. The greater the force, the greater the acceleration (where mass is constant). However, a change in mass will affect the acceleration. As mass increases, the rate of acceleration will decrease, but as mass decreases, the rate of acceleration will increase.

As an athlete pushes off the starting block, his rate of acceleration will be directly proportional to the force he exerts. If he repeats the push off but applies twice as much force, he will double the rate of acceleration. A runner can therefore increase his acceleration by increasing the force he applies backward and downward against the running surface. Because acceleration is inversely proportional to mass, if the runner loses weight then acceleration would increase for the same force. If he gains weight, acceleration will decrease for the same force. A swimmer will increase acceleration by increasing the force applied by his arms and legs against the water; if he loses weight, he will travel faster using the same effort.

Maximum acceleration will be achieved when all the contributing forces are directed in the line of desired movement, applied maximally in the appropriate sequence and with correct timing.

Muscle contraction provides the forces which increase acceleration (the stronger the muscles, the greater the force they can generate). The more forceful the contraction, the more energy is expended. This has implications in endurance activities such as long distance running where energy must be conserved, and so the rate of acceleration must be carefully considered.

The third law – applied to sport

The third law (the law of counterforce) explains that every action will generate a reaction which is equal and opposite to it. A force applied to a stable surface will produce an equal force in the opposite direction.

When the foot exerts a force against a firm surface, an equal and opposite force is returned from the surface. This push back from the surface produces a force which propels the body in the direction of the force. The greater the force applied by the foot, the greater the reaction force and the greater the propulsion and acceleration. If the surface is slippery or is soft, then the reaction force is dissipated and reduced.

These opposing forces can cause problems for athletes during hard training, as the constant jarring from reaction forces as the feet strike the ground, can cause repetitive stress injuries such as shin splints and spinal problems. Training should take place on appropriate surfaces, and correct, well manufactured footwear with cushioned soles should be worn to dissipate forces. Exercising should be performed in a gymnasium or hall with a sprung floor to reduce the risk of injury.

Gravity

This is the force which attracts or pulls all objects towards the earth; it is a continual, vertical, downward force. This gravitational force provides the weight of an object, which varies in different locations, depending on the force of the gravitational field (remember that the *mass* of the object always remains the same). On the surface of the moon where the pull is weak, weight is greatly reduced. However, on the earth's surface the gravitational field exerts a force of approximately 10 Newtons for every Kilogram of mass, whether the object is on the ground or a projectile in the air.

Once a projectile or an athlete produces an upward thrust and breaks contact with the surface, the force of gravity acts to pull him back down. The greater the mass, the greater the gravitational force acting on it. Gravitational pull affects most body movement – it will *assist* movement in the same direction but *resist* movement in the opposite direction. It is an important consideration when planning exercises. Movements performed downward with gravity will involve different muscle work from those performed upwards against gravity.

The centre of gravity

This is an imaginary point at the centre of a body or mass through which its weight is said to act, or around which it is perfectly balanced. In the standing position, the centre of gravity of the human body lies approximately at the second sacral vertebra, but this will vary with the shape and weight distribution of the individual. More weight on the top half of the body (the chest and shoulders) will raise the centre of gravity, whereas more weight on the lower half (the hips and thighs) will lower it.

The lower the centre of gravity, the more stable the object, therefore a person with more weight distributed around the hips and thighs is relatively more stable than a person with more weight around the chest and arms. It is an advantage in some sports such as the high jump to have a high centre of gravity, but it is a disadvantage in sports that require stability such as wrestling.

Anti gravity muscles

The upright posture is maintained by particular muscle groups known as postural muscles or anti gravity muscles. They must work continuously to oppose the pull of gravity and keep the body upright. If posture is good and the body perfectly balanced, the effort for these muscles is minimal. Poor posture occurs when segments move out of alignment, which will alter the balance and increase the effort required from certain muscle groups. This imbalance will result in the shortening of some muscles and the stretching and weakening of others.

Regular exercise of the large muscle groups will maintain muscle strength and balance, thus preventing abnormal postures. If deformities have developed, specific exercises must be practised to stretch the shortened muscles and strengthen the weak muscles.

The anti gravity muscles are:

- anterior tibials
- posterior tibials
- quadriceps
- hip extensors
- errector spinae
- abdominals

- trapezius and the rhomboids
- neck extensors
- neck flexors.

The line of gravity

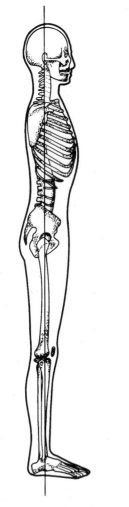

This is an imaginary line which falls perpendicularly (vertically) through the centre of gravity and through which the force of gravity acts. The line of gravity of the human body passes through the vertex (top of the head), through the mid cervical vertebrae, in front of the thoracic vertebrae, behind the bodies of the lumbar vertebrae, through the second sacral vertebra, slightly in front of the knee joint, in front of the ankle joint, ending between the ball of the foot and the heel.

The line of gravity is a useful measure when examining posture. When the body adopts the correct posture, a line in the same plane but lateral to the line of gravity will fall through the lobe of the ear, the point of the shoulder (ie, the acromion process) through the hip joint, to the front of the knee joint but behind the patella, in front of the ankle joint and ending between the ball of the foot and the heel.

Figure 5.1   *The line of gravity*

Base

The base of an object is the area of contact with the surface. Any object with two or more parts on the ground, will have a base which includes the area of the parts and the space in between. In standing positions, the feet will be in contact with the surface; during handstands the hands will be in contact. In sitting, the base includes the feet and the area

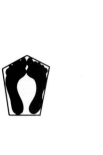 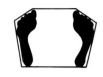

Figure 5.2 *The size of the base*

between the legs of the chair; in lying, the area of the body surface on the ground is the base.

Stability

Stability means that a body is firmly balanced, and will not easily fall over.

The stability of a body depends on the relationship between the centre of gravity and line of gravity with the base. Stability is greatest when the centre of gravity is directly over the centre of the base. As the centre of gravity moves towards the edge of the base, the object becomes increasingly unstable. If the centre and line of gravity fall outside the base, the body is unbalanced in that direction, and the body will fall over unless a quick action is taken to regain balance. This will require an adjustment of the body parts, either to enlarge the base, or to move the centre of gravity back towards the centre of the base.

- Balancing skills involve constant minor adjustments to return the centre of gravity over the base or to enlarge the base.

Standing with a small base is less stable than standing with a large base; eg, if a person stands with the feet together, the base is relatively small (the area of the feet). Therefore, if the body moves forward, sideways or backwards without adjusting the position of the feet, the line of gravity will easily fall outside the base and the body will fall over. A quick movement of the foot in the direction of the imbalance will restore balance and prevent this happening. Standing with the feet apart, ie, stride standing, will increase the size of the base, which is now the area of the feet and the area between. When the body moves, the line of gravity will more easily remain within the base and the body will not easily fall over. Exercises or movements of the arms and trunks are easier to perform in stride standing, when the body is more stable.

The body is given maximum stability when lying on the ground, as there is a large base and low centre of gravity.

Factors which influence stability are:

- the position of the centre of gravity: the lower the centre of gravity, the greater the stability
- the size of the base: the larger the base, the greater the stability
- the mass of the body: the greater the mass of the body, the greater the stability
- friction between feet and the ground (increases stability)
- focusing vision on a stationary object (increases stability).

Levers

A lever is a rigid bar which revolves around a pivot or fixed point known as the fulcrum. We are all familiar with the use of a lever to prise the lid off a tin of paint. When a coin is placed under the lid, and a force applied on the other side, the lid lifts up. If the coin does not work, we use a spoon handle or some longer rigid bar, and this will more easily lift the lid because it has greater mechanical advantage. The principles of leverage also apply to body movement, which occurs as a result of the actions of body levers.

The components of a lever are:

1 rigid bar
2 fulcrum (F)
3 effort (E)
4 weight (W) (this may also be termed load or resistance).

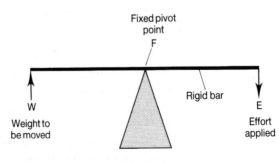

Figure 5.3 *A lever*

The *rigid bar* moves about a fixed point called the *fulcrum*. A force or *effort* applied at one point on the lever moves a second force or *weight* (resistance) applied at another point.

The distance between the point where the effort is applied and the fulcrum is known as the *effort arm* (EA), and the distance from the point of application of the weight to the fulcrum is known as the *weight arm* (WA).

- When E × EA = W × WA, there is no movement and the lever is balanced.
- If E × EA is greater than W × WA, movement will occur in the direction of the effort.
- If W × WA is greater than E × EA, movement occurs in the direction of the weight.

In the human body:

- The bones are the rigid bar.
- The joint is the fulcrum.
- The effort is the pull of the contracting muscle or muscles at their point of insertion.
- The weight is the body part being moved.

There are *three* different types, classes or orders of levers. They are different because of the position of the fulcrum in relation to the effort and the weight.

First order of lever (EFW)

In the first order, the fulcrum (F) lies between the effort (E) and the weight (W). The fulcrum may be nearer the weight (thereby giving a longer effort arm) or may lie nearer the effort (giving a longer weight arm). When the effort arm is longer than the weight arm, less effort is required, and there is mechanical advantage. If the weight arm is longer than the effort arm, more effort is required, and there is mechanical disadvantage.

We find examples of this first order in everyday life, but few in the body:

- A see-saw has a rigid bar which moves around a fulcrum. When two people sit on a see-saw, the heavier of the two has to sit nearer the fulcrum; if they sit an equal distance from the fulcrum, the lever will move down on the side of the heavier weight.
- During the extension of the head, the fulcrum lies at the cervical joints. The effort is supplied by the muscle pull at

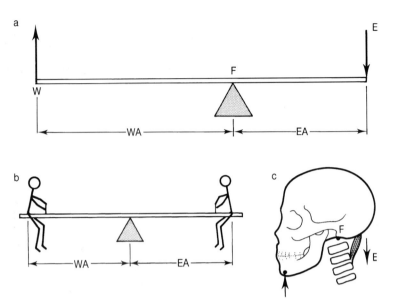

Figure 5.4 *The first order of levers*

the point of insertion, and the weight is the head being moved. In order to move the head backwards, the muscle power and the distance from the fulcrum must be greater than the weight of the head and its distance from the fulcrum.

Second order of lever (FWE)

In this order, the weight lies between the fulcrum and the effort. The effort arm will always be longer than the weight arm, and as less effort is required to move the lever, there will always be mechanical advantage. This is a lever capable of moving a large weight over a short distance at slow speed.

Examples are found in everyday life and in the body where power is needed:

■ A wheelbarrow has the fulcrum at the wheel, the weight in the middle and the effort at the handle. Because the effort arm is always longer than the weight arm, it is quite easy to lift a heavy load in a wheelbarrow.

■ When raising the heel off the ground, the fulcrum is at the metatarso-phalangeal joints, the body weight falls down the leg to the ankle, and the effort to lift the heel is from the plantar flexors (gastrocnemeus and soleus) at their point of insertion. When these muscles contract, they are able to lift a considerable amount of body weight

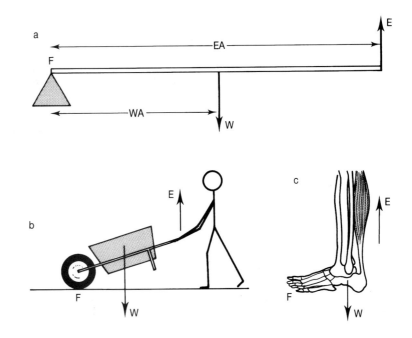

Figure 5.5 *The second order of levers*

because of the long effort arm compared with the weight arm.

Third order of lever (FEW)

In this order the effort lies between the fulcrum and the weight. The effort arm will always be shorter than the weight arm; the shorter the effort arm, the more effort is required to move the lever. Therefore this will be a lever of mechanical disadvantage, but a long resistance arm with a short effort arm will produce movement at greater speed and distance.

Examples are found in everyday life, and this is the most common type of leverage found in the body:

- Tongs for picking up objects have the fulcrum at one end, the effort is applied in the middle and the weight lies at the other end.
- During flexion of the elbow to lift the forearm, the fulcrum lies at the elbow joint. The effort is applied at the point of insertion of biceps and brachialis, and the weight is the arm being lifted plus any weight in the hand. Here the effort arm is short and the weight arm is long, and much effort is required to move the weight, but

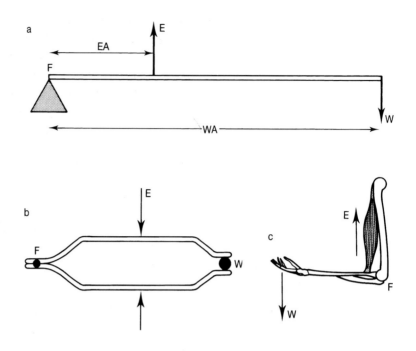

Figure 5.6 *The third order of levers*

the long lever will produce a large range and speed. It is an advantage for runners and jumpers to have long limbs for speed and range.

Leverage related to muscle work

The third order of lever produces movement of great range and speed in the body. If the fulcrum is the joint where movement is taking place, the effort is provided by the muscle power exerted when the muscle contracts; the effort arm is the distance from the joint to the point where the muscle inserts (this cannot be changed); the weight is the part being moved (which can be increased by adding weight to the part); and the weight arm is the distance from the fulcrum to the end of the moving part (this can be shortened by flexing joints, or increased by adding length, eg, a pole or dumb bell). Therefore, we can increase the effort for the muscle by increasing the weight or lengthening the weight arm.

If the muscle strength × effort arm is greater than weight × weight arm, movement will occur. If we then increase the weight, or the length of the weight arm, greater muscle strength will be required to produce movement; this principle is used to strengthen muscles:

■ if the maximum weight that a muscle can lift is identified, the muscle is made to lift just less than this weight a set number of times. When the muscle strengthens and is able to lift the weight 30 times, the weight is increased. Over a period of time, the muscle becomes stronger as the weight is progressively increased (see Chapter 7).

EXAMPLES OF EXERCISES TO STRENGTHEN MUSCLES

1 Increasing the work to strengthen *abdominal* muscles:
   Crook lying:
   A arms across chest, curl up (short weight arm)
   B hands on ears, curl up (longer weight arm)
   C arms stretch above head, curl up (longer weight arm)
   D arms across chest holding weight, curl up (increased weight)
   E arms stretch above head holding weight, curl up (increased weight arm and weight)

This progression continues by increasing the weight to be lifted. Once the muscle can lift the weight 10 × 3 times, the weight can be increased.

2 Increasing the work to strengthen *deltoid*:
   Stride standing:
   A hand on shoulder, lift arm sideways (short weight arm)
   B hand to side, lift arm sideways (longer weight arm)
   C hand to side holding pole, lift arm sideways (longer weight arm)
   D hand to side holding weight, lift arm sideways (increased weight). This weight can be increased as the muscle gets stronger
   E hand to side holding weight at the end of the pole, lift arm sideways (longer weight arm and increased weight).

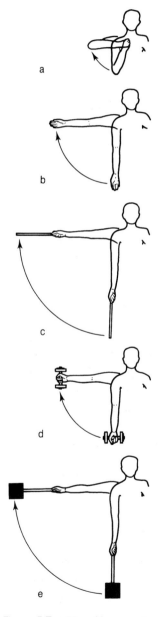

a

b

c

d

e

Figure 5.7 *Use of leverage to progress exercise*

Questions

1 Explain the difference between the *mass* of an object, and the *weight* of an object.

2 Define the following terms:
- acceleration
- impetus
- inertia.

3 Define the terms *gravity* and *centre of gravity*.

4 Where is the approximate position of the centre of gravity in the human body?

5 When assessing posture, list the points for identification through which the line of gravity will fall.

6 Complete the following:
The base of an object is that part which ....

7 Give any three factors which influence the stability of a body.

8 Explain why it is preferable to exercise on a sprung floor.

9 Draw three diagrams to illustrate the three classes of levers.

10 Relate the parts of a lever to the human body.

11 Give two ways in which leverage can be used to increase the resistance to muscle work.

12 Show two ways of using leverage to make the following exercise harder for the *gluteus maximus*:
prone lying, raise the leg off the floor, knee bent to right angle.

CHAPTER 6

Concepts of Movement

Muscles work to produce or control movement at joints. When a muscle is working, tension builds up within it; the muscle may shorten, lengthen or remain the same length, depending on the action required.

A muscle may be required to move a part, to control the effect of an external force or to hold a specific static position. Each of these actions will require a different type of muscle contraction. Movements also vary in degree and complexity and may be required to contact through their full range of movement, ie, from full stretch to full contraction, or through only a part of this range. Many muscles must work together as a group to bring about smooth, co-ordinated movement. All the muscles around the moving joint have a specific role to play. This chapter explains these concepts and teaches the student to analyse movement.

Types of muscle work

The type of work will depend on what the muscle is required to do:

- if the muscle is required to move a part, it will shorten (concentric work)
- when required to control the effect of an external force, the muscle will lengthen (eccentric work)
- if it is required to hold or stabilise a specific position, it remains the same length (static work).

Muscle work is classified into two main types: *isotonic* and *isometric*.

Isotonic muscle work

Isotonic means equal tone: the muscle changes in length throughout the movement, but the tone remains the same. The muscle may shorten during *concentric* work, or may lengthen during *eccentric* work.

In practice, it is difficult for tone to remain constant throughout full range movement because of the difference in the angle of pull of the muscle. Special machines which automatically adjust the resistance may be used to keep muscle tension constant throughout the range. This is an excellent method of strength training for those athletes needing strength in full and outer range. This is known as *isokinetic* work.

Concentric work (isotonic shortening or positive phase)

A muscle working concentrically shortens and thickens, the origin and insertion move towards each other and movement is produced in the joint; eg, bending the elbow to lift a weight is concentric work for the elbow flexors, because they shorten to flex the elbow.

Concentric muscle work is generally the most effective for muscle strengthening, although eccentric and static work should also be included.

Eccentric muscle work (isotonic lengthening or negative phase)

A muscle working eccentrically becomes longer and thinner, as the origin and insertion move away from each other. The muscle pays out gradually to control the movement produced by some external force such as gravity, springs etc.; eg, when lowering the weight back down, the elbow flexors lengthen and pay out gradually to lower it smoothly downwards.

Eccentric muscle work can sometimes be easier to perform but produces muscle soreness. It is useful when re-

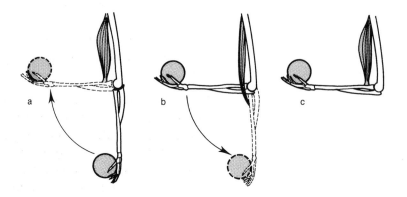

Figure 6.1   *Types of muscle work: the biceps working (a) concentrically (b) eccentrically (c) statically to hold the ball*

educating muscles if they cannot perform concentric work. Eccentric work in full and outer range maintains flexibility. Power lifters use negative repetitions with weights too great for concentric contraction: spotters lift the weight into position and the lifter lowers it.

Isometric muscle work (static)

Isometric means equal length: the length of the muscle does not change but there is a change in tone. Tension within the muscle increases but there is no joint movement. Isometric work is also known as *static* work.

A muscle working statically does not change in length but there is an increase in muscle tone. The origin and insertion do not move and there is no joint movement; eg, holding the weight mid-way means that the elbow flexors have to increase in tone to maintain the position, but there is no movement at the elbow joint. Muscles can be made to work statically by pushing against immovable objects or holding against heavy weights or springs. When used for muscle strengthening, static contractions should be performed at different points throughout the range.

Static work is easy to perform but muscles fatigue quickly. This is because of the constant compression on the blood vessels and capillary networks which impedes blood flow. This limits the delivery of oxygen and nutrients and removal of waste products. Static work should be practised for short periods with frequent rest intervals.

Static work increases blood pressure and should not be performed by those with heart and blood pressure problems.

Range of movement

When muscles contract, they move the joint through a certain range. There are four ranges that a muscle or joint can work through:

1 *Full range* – from full stretch to full contraction. This is rarely used under normal activities, but is essential for maintaining full joint mobility and muscle flexibility, and is useful for reducing tension.
2 *Outer range* – from full stretch to mid point of contraction. This is difficult due to the angle of pull of

the muscle, and energy is wasted in compression of joint surfaces (shunting). However, exercises in both full and outer ranges prevent shortening of the muscles and maintain joint mobility. Outer range is used for stretching/flexibility work.

3 *Inner range* – from full contraction to mid point. This is used when re-educating weak muscles and for strengthening work, as the angle of pull is advantageous.

4 *Middle range* – any distance from mid point of outer to mid point of inner. This is the range in which muscles are most often used in everyday activities. They are more efficient in this range because the angle of pull of the muscle is nearer 90°, but full joint movement is never achieved in this range.

The group action of muscles

When muscles contract to produce movement, they work in groups. Each member of the group has a particular role to play, rather like the members of an orchestra. They work together in a synchronised manner to produce smooth, co-ordinated, efficient movement.

There are four different members which are named according to their function. They are the:

- agonists or prime movers
- antagonists
- synergists
- fixators.

1 *The agonists or prime movers* – These are the muscles which contract to produce the required movement (prime action).

For example: abduction of the hip joint is produced by the abductors, therefore gluteus medius, gluteus minimus and tensor fascia lata are the agonists or prime movers.

2 *The antagonists* – These lie on the opposite side of the joint from the agonists. They must relax and lengthen in a controlled manner so that the movement produced by the agonists is performed smoothly.

For example: when the abductors are contracting to abduct the hip joint, the opposite group (the adductors) must relax. Therefore adductors magnus, longus, brevis, pectineus and gracilis are the antagonists.

3 *The synergists* – These muscles assist the prime movers to produce the most efficient movement. They may alter the angle of pull of the prime mover, or prevent unwanted movement.

For example: during abduction of the hip, the deep hip muscles work isometrically to prevent the hip rotating so that maximum effort is put into abduction. Therefore piriformis and the obturator muscles are the synergists.

4 *The fixators* – These muscles ensure that the prime movers act from a fixed base. They stabilise and prevent unnecessary movements in surrounding joints.

For example: during abduction of the hip joint, the pelvis is held steady. Therefore the trunk side flexors and abductors of the opposite side work statically to fix the pelvis, and are the fixators.

Balance between muscle groups

The agonists and antagonists are the most vital members of the group and require identification when analysing muscle work. When the agonists are contracting to produce movement, the antagonists must relax to allow the movement to take place. This is controlled by the nervous system and is known as *reciprocal relaxation*. This is used in certain stretching techniques. It is sufficient to remember that while synergists and fixators are also contributing to the movement, their identification is difficult and unnecessary.

Muscles can change their role within a group depending on the movement. The patterns of movement are initiated and synchronised in the motor cortex of the brain, and the appropriate impulses are conveyed to the muscles via their motor nerves.

The muscles acting on a joint are arranged around the joint; some are superficial while others are deep. The agonists and antagonists are arranged as opposite pairs – flexors opposite extensors, abductors opposite adductors, medial rotators opposite lateral rotators. When the flexors are the agonists, the extensors will be the antagonists and vice versa (other smaller muscles will be synergists and fixators).

The balance between agonists and antagonists is very important, as tightness and shortening or over stretching and weakness of one group, will affect the function of the other, preventing full range movement and limiting athletic performance. Stresses will be imposed on the underlying joints and ligaments which may result in deformity and pain. Exercises and training must always be planned to maintain balance between agonists and antagonists.

Analysis of muscle work for exercise schemes

All exercise schemes require careful planning to ensure that the set objectives are realised. For corrective schemes or training routines, the exercises must be carefully planned to target specific muscles or groups; some will require strengthening, while others require stretching. For general schemes, all the main muscle groups must be included and balance maintained between opposing muscles.

Planning exercise schemes therefore requires the ability to analyse the muscle work. This procedure should be followed:

- Give the starting position (to determine the effect of gravity on the movement), eg, lying, stride standing
- Name the moving joint, eg, hip, shoulder
- Name the direction of movement, eg, flexion, abduction
- Name the prime movers, ie, the muscles producing the movement
- Name the type of muscle work, ie, concentric, eccentric or static
- Name the range of movement, ie, inner, outer, middle or full.

Identifying the type of muscle work poses the greatest difficulty for most students. **Remember:**

- If the muscle is shortening and the origin and insertion are moving nearer to each other, the work is *concentric*.
- If the movement is produced by an external force such as gravity, weights, springs etc., the muscle is lengthening and paying out to control the movement, and the origin and insertion are moving away from each other, the work is *eccentric*.
- If the muscle is contracting but producing no movement at the joint, the work is *static*.

Sample analyses of muscle work

Exercises performed in different starting positions will have different muscle work; eg, abduction and adduction of the hip joint performed in different positions.

Example 1:
- Lying, part legs
- Moving joint: hip
- Direction of move: abduction
- Prime movers: the abductors (gluteus medius, minimus and tensor fasiae latae)
- Muscle work: concentric (muscle shortens producing the movement)
- Range: inner

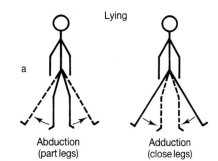

Figure 6.2 *Abduction and adduction of the legs (a) lying*

Example 2:
- Lying, close legs
- Moving joint: hip
- Direction of move: adduction
- Prime movers: adductors (adductor longus, magnus, brevis, pectineus, gracilis)
- Muscle work: concentric
- Range: outer

In the lying position when the legs are opened and closed, gravity is not affecting the movement since gravitational

Side lying

Abduction
(leg raise)

b

Adduction
(leg lower)

(b) side lying

pull is downwards, but the movement is in the *horizontal* plane. Both the abductors and adductors work concentrically.

Now if we change the starting position but do the same movement the muscle work changes.

Example 3:
- Side lying, upper leg raise
- Moving joint: hip joint
- Direction of move: abduction
- Prime movers: abductors (as before)
- Muscle work: concentric (muscle shortens)
- Range: inner

(This movement is against the pull of gravity.)

Example 4:
- Side lying, leg lowering
  (Gravity would pull the leg down, therefore the muscle work changes as we do not need the adductors to work.)
- Moving joint: hip joint
- Direction of move: adduction
- Prime movers: abductors (because gravity will pull leg down)
- Muscle work: eccentric
- Range: inner

Only the abductors work in this position, first concentrically and then eccentrically.

If we change the starting position yet again, the muscle work will change again.

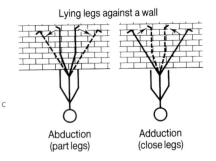

Lying legs against a wall

c

Abduction (part legs)   Adduction (close legs)

(c) lying with legs against a wall

Example 5:
- Lying with legs at right angles against a wall, part legs
- Moving joint: hip joint
- Direction of move: abduction
- Prime movers: adductors (because gravity will put legs out)

- Muscle work: eccentric
- Range: outer

Example 6:
- Lying with legs at right angles against a wall, close legs
- Moving joint: hip joint
- Direction of move: adduction
- Prime movers: adductors
- Muscle work: concentric
- Range: outer

Only the adductors work in this position, first eccentrically and then concentrically.

Now work out the muscle work of elbow flexion and extension in the following starting positions (Remember that biceps flexes the elbow and triceps extends the elbow.):

1 Stride standing (arms at side) – raise hand to touch shoulder.
2 As above – lower hand back down.
3 Yard stride standing – bring hand in to touch shoulder.
4 As above – bring hand back out to yard.
5 Head rest stride standing – raise hand up to elevation.
6 As above – lower hand back to head.

The classification of movement

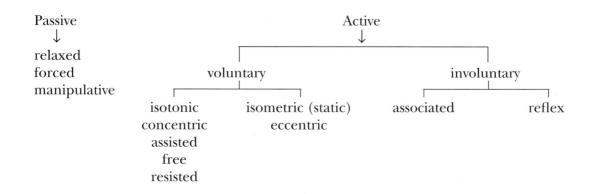

Figure 6.3 *Classifications of movement*

Passive movements

These movements are performed by an external force when the client's own muscles are inactive (ie, do not contract). The therapist moves the joint but the client plays no active part. These movements are used to maintain or increase the mobility in joints.

They may be classified into:

1 *Relaxed passive movements* – performed within the existing range. These movements are used to maintain joint mobility when the client's muscles are unable to contract due to injury, paralysis, etc.
2 *Forced passive movements* – performed beyond the existing range. These are used to increase the range of movement at joints. They are included in some flexibility training schemes, when a partner exerts pressure at the end of the range to gain more movement and stretch. They must only be performed by trained therapists with complete knowledge of joint function.
3 *Manipulative passive movements* – these are forced movements performed under anaesthetic, and are carried out to break down adhesions which are limiting joint movement. They must only be carried out by medical practitioners/consultants.

Active movements

These may be voluntary (ie, under the control of the will) or involuntary (ie, not under the control of the will). They may be categorised as:

1 *Involuntary movements* – not controlled by the will and may be:
    A reflex movements such as blinking or movement away from hot or painful conditions
    B associated movements which are done by the fixators and synergists during active movements.
2 *Voluntary movements* – controlled by the will, the result of voluntary action of muscles. They may be isotonic or isometric:

Concentric movements may be further subdivided into assisted, free and resisted:

■ Assisted active exercise – When muscle power is

inadequate to produce a desired movement, its power can be helped by the use of an external force acting with the muscle pull. The movement is thus assisted.

- Free active exercise – This is movement where the working muscles are subjected only to the forces of gravity acting upon the part being moved.
- Resisted active exercise – This is movement where the action of the muscles is resisted by an external force, eg, weights, springs, water etc. This resistance acts against the muscle pull, and can be increased progressively to develop muscle power and endurance.

Questions

1 Give the two main types of muscle work.
2 Define the terms *concentric work* and *eccentric work*, and give one example of each.
3 Explain the four ranges of movement.
4 Name each member which contributes to the group action of muscles.
5 Define the terms
   - Prime mover – agonist
   - Antagonist
6 List the points to consider when analysing muscle work.

7 Analyse the muscle work of the following actions:
Stride standing:
   - Raise the arm out to the side to shoulder level
   - Lower the arm back down to the side
Analyse these movements when the body is in supine lying.
8 Define the terms *active movement* and *passive movement*.

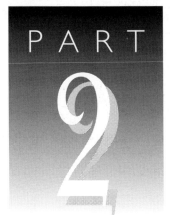

PART

2

Training for Fitness

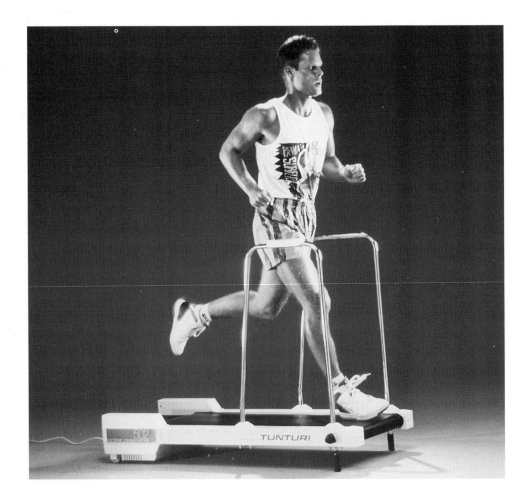

CHAPTER 7

Fitness Training

Fitness means having enough energy and skill to cope in one's environment. The fitness levels required by individuals will vary greatly, from the lowest level required by the infirm just to cope with daily living, to the optimum fitness required by top elite athletes and sports people. All age groups can improve their fitness level through regular exercise, providing the exercises begin at the appropriate level, progress gradually and allow adequate time for recovery.

Although fitness and health are inter-related, it is important to distinguish between the two. Health may be defined as 'freedom from disease'. It is therefore possible to be healthy, but unfit; it is also possible to be superbly fit and compete at the highest level while suffering from ill health such as colds, infections, etc. However, one's state of health can affect and limit performance. In the same way as the body must be allowed time to recover from intense activity, it must be allowed time to recover from disease. If it is necessary and possible to continue training when suffering from disease, the intensity of training must be decreased to maintenance levels.

How to improve fitness

Improving fitness means improving the physiological functioning of various body systems. To achieve this, the body must be encouraged to work harder than it normally has to. This is done by overloading the systems through exercises or activities which become progressively more demanding. The systems adapt in response to these additional stresses and become more efficient. As soon as the body copes with one level of stress, the overload must increase. The process is repeated until the desired level of fitness is achieved. In this way, the body is *trained* to deal with increasing workload.

When the desired fitness level is achieved, training will continue at this level of intensity or just above to maintain the training effect. It is important to remember that the overload applied must be appropriate to the individual, and must progress gradually; too much overload applied too rapidly will result in breakdown and damage.

Training principles

The fitness trainer must fully understand the following principles, as they apply to all conditioning programmes, regardless of which systems are to be improved.

Specificity

This means that the exercises/overload, must be specific to those muscles or energy systems targeted for conditioning. This is because training effects are generally not transferable; eg, strength training will not improve endurance, and vice versa.

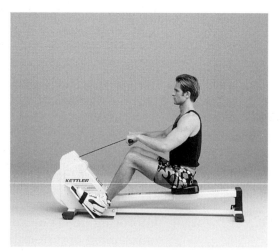

Figure 7.1   *Fitness training*

Training threshold

This refers to the minimum intensity of exercise required to bring about an improvement; eg, to improve cardio-vascular endurance, an individual must exercise at 60–80% of maximum heart rate (MHR) for 20–30 minutes three times per week. 60% indicates the minimum intensity, which must increase as fitness develops. For strength training, overload must be at least 66% of 1 RM (one repetition maximum) and increased as strength develops.

Overload

This means that the appropriate systems are stressed beyond normal requirements. Overload may be adjusted by changing the intensity, frequency and/or duration, and must always be appropriate to the fitness level of the individual. Too little will not produce a training effect; too much can cause damage. Overload must increase as fitness develops.

Progression

This means that the exercises must become progressively harder to increase fitness levels. This may be achieved by increasing intensity, frequency or duration.

Intensity

This indicates how hard the body is working; eg, for aerobic fitness, the individual must exercise at an intensity of 60–90% of MHR. Beginners will start at 60%, and will gradually increase as fitness develops, to 85 or 90%. For muscle strength, intensity refers to the amount of weight lifted.

Duration

This is the length of time of the exercise session. The longer the session, the more exercises will be performed. This will increase with fitness.

Frequency

This refers to the number of training sessions per week. Two to three sessions is the minimum recommended, but three to four sessions per week will result in greater improvement. Elite athletes may include some form of training every day. They may train different muscles or systems, allowing recovery time for others. Exercises must be performed on a regular basis or training effects are lost.

Reversibility

This refers to the loss of training effect if an individual stops exercising. Training effect may be lost within just two weeks and there will be a considerable loss of fitness after a period of four to six weeks after training stops. Decline in fitness is slower in those who have trained over a long period of time.

The components of fitness

The essential types of fitness for athletes and sportspeople are generally thought of as:

- strength
- stamina
- flexibility
- speed.

Individuals may require more of one than another, depending on the demands of their sport; eg, weight lifters require muscle strength, marathon runners require stamina, ballet dancers require flexibility, sprinters require speed. Each of these components can be specifically trained, but most sports require more than one.

To improve fitness, we must improve the following components:

- Cardio-respiratory endurance (aerobic endurance)
- Muscle strength
- Muscle endurance
- Flexibility
- Body composition

In addition to improving these physical components, one must include:

- speed
- skill (including co-ordination, balance, timing, rhythm, agility)

Finally, total fitness must also give consideration to:

- nutrition (ie, diet)
- rest and relaxation.

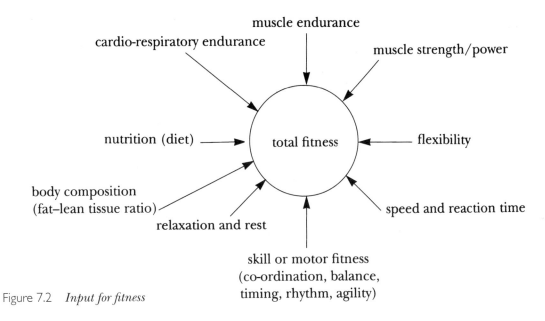

Figure 7.2   *Input for fitness*

1 Explain what is meant by each of the following terms
   A Training threshold
   B Overload
   C Reversibility
2 List the three variables which may be increased to ensure progression during fitness training.

3 List four components of fitness.
4 Explain why overload must be gradually applied.
5 Discuss the difference between 'health' and 'fitness'.
6 Explain why exercise must be appropriate to the level of fitness of the individual.

CHAPTER 8

Cardio-Respiratory Endurance

Cardio-vascular/cardio-pulmonary fitness, aerobic fitness and endurance fitness all mean the same thing; these terms refer to the efficiency of the lungs to take in oxygen and remove carbon dioxide, the efficiency of the heart and circulation to transport oxygen to the contracting muscles, and the muscle's ability to utilise the oxygen. An individual's capacity to exercise without fatigue is dependent on these factors.

Before exercise, the body is in a balanced state known as *homeostasis*, and the systems just meet the body's metabolic needs. When exercise begins, the systems must respond rapidly to the increased demand for nutrients and oxygen (required to produce ATP, the energy source for muscle contraction). Ventilation in the lungs must increase and breathing becomes faster and deeper. Cardiac output must increase, therefore heart rate and stroke volume must increase.

Improving cardio-respiratory endurance

Training methods and techniques

Training can increase the capacity of the lungs to take in oxygen and efficiency of the heart/vascular system to deliver oxygen. The utilisation of oxygen within muscle tissue will improve because haemoglobin levels rise, and the mitochondria (energy producers) within the cells increase in size and number. Therefore with appropriate training, the capacity to exercise aerobically will increase.

Any form of low intensity, long duration activity regularly performed will improve endurance, providing the effort is above the training threshold. These activities include:

- running
- jogging
- swimming
- walking
- cross-country skiing
- skating
- cycling
- aerobic dance or exercise programmes
- treadmill walking.

The activity that provides greatest satisfaction and enjoyment is usually the most successful, as motivation is enhanced. The principles of training outlined on page 116 will apply to any of the above activities.

A minimum amount of exercise must be performed to produce a training effect; for aerobic conditioning, the overload must be selected according to the fitness level of the individual and increased gradually as fitness improves. This is done in three ways:

1 Increasing the *intensity* of exercise – making the exercises harder.
2 Increasing the *duration* of exercise – performing the exercises for a longer time.
3 Increasing the *frequency* of exercise – performing the exercises more often.

Intensity

Increasing the intensity is one way of making the body work progressively harder. Research indicates that intensity has the greatest effect on improving aerobic capacity. The heart rate is an excellent indicator of how hard the body is working.

HEART RATE

The heart rate is the same as the pulse rate and can be taken at pulse points throughout the body. The usual point for reading pulse rate is at the wrist (the radial pulse point).

Average heart rate of the adult male is around 72–76 beats/minute, and the average adult female is around 76–80 beats/minute.

MAXIMUM HEART RATE (MHR)

Maximum heart rate (MHR) is the rate at near exhaustion. Exercising at this rate would be inadvisable as it will produce a dangerous level of stress, so individuals should keep below their maximum heart rate when exercising. Aerobic capacity will improve if the exercising heart rate is maintained between 70% and 90% of MHR. This is referred to as the *aerobic training zone.*

To calculate an average person's maximal heart rate, deduct the person's age from 220.

■ eg, the maximum heart rate for a 40 year old person will be 220 − 40 = 180 beats/minute.

The unfit should begin exercising at 60% of MHR but move into the training zone of 70% and over as fitness improves. The very fit may exercise at up to 90% of MHR.

For a 40 year old person, 60% of MHR will be:

$$0.60 \times 180 = 108 \text{ beats/min}$$

OR you can work it out this way:

$$180 \times \frac{60}{100} = 108 \text{ beats/min (this is the target heart rate)}$$

This person should exercise with sufficient intensity to maintain a pulse rate of 108 beats per minute for 20–30 minutes duration, two to three times per week.

After four to six weeks, it will be safe to exercise at 70% of maximum heart rate; ie

$$0.70 \times 180 = 126 \text{ beats/min}$$

OR

$$180 \times \frac{70}{100} = 126 \text{ beats/min (target rate)}$$

Eventually, as fitness increases, he may exercise at 80% or 90% of MHR.

Duration

This is the actual time that a person is exercising at the target heart rate, and may last for 15–30 minutes or more depending on fitness level. It does not include the warm up and cool down. This is the main phase of an exercise session, and will involve the large muscle groups – it is known as the *conditioning phase*. The session will begin with a warm up phase of 15–20 minutes (this will include stretch), followed by the 15–30 minute conditioning phase (exercising at target heart rate), and will end with a 5–10 minute cool down.

Frequency

This is the number of sessions per week which may vary from two to three times for an unfit beginner, up to four to five times as fitness improves. Many top athletes train every day.

Any single or combination of the three variables may be increased as fitness develops, to maintain training effects in any aerobic activity. Increasing intensity is essential to the development of fitness.

Dangers of aerobic activities

- Repetitive stress injuries mainly of ankle, knees, back and shins ie, (shin splints).
- Dehydration.

Running

Different forms of running are used to improve aerobic capacity. Running can be used to improve both aerobic and anaerobic systems:

- Slow running or jogging, involving low effort over a period of time when breathing is easy, will improve aerobic systems.
- Fast running or sprinting, resulting in breathlessness, will improve anaerobic systems.

Athletes frequently combine these forms of running and other specific exercise routines in their training programmes.

Long continuous running or slow distance running

This uses low level effort over a long period of time. This form of training is suitable for those beginning a fitness programme, and also for those wanting to reduce body fat. Middle distance runners may use this form of training as it is almost the same as competition. Marathon runners may use it, but at a slower pace as a greater distance must be covered. To dictate the pace:

- assess fitness
- calculate MHR
- run at target heart rate 70%–80% of MHR for a certain distance in a set period of time (around 30 minutes).

This can be varied by keeping the same distance, but decreasing the time (faster pace), then increasing the distance in the original time, and so on. This develops aerobic endurance, and trains the body to use fatty acids as fuel, but does not develop speed or power.

Varied pace running (Swedish Fartlek running)

This varies the pace at specific intervals throughout the run. Continuous steady pace running or fast striding is interrupted at intervals by quick sprints. This will combine both anaerobic and aerobic energy systems and is a more realistic training for most sports. It can be varied to use only aerobic systems if low effort is used in all stages.

It may involve running over different terrain, through forests, fields, uphill, downhill on sand, gravel and grass. Tracks are very carefully graded for degree of difficulty. This type of speed play programme may include:

- 10–15 mins jogging
- 5 mins rapid walk
- 1 mile slow distance running
- 10 mins rapid walk
- 10 mins jogging.

The variations in pace can be selected to mirror closely the demands of a particular sport or activity.

Interval training

This is a method where a set period of effort is followed by a set recovery phase. It can involve a 30 second period of fast running, sufficient to raise the pulse rate to 180 bpm, followed by a 90 second recovery period of slow jogging. This is performed over a measured distance of between 150–300 metres. The sequence is repeated 6–10 times.

The light work period allows the oxygen debt incurred during the fast work period to be repaid. This method will improve both aerobic and anaerobic systems. Again, the intensity, recovery time and rest interval can be adjusted to suit the individual.

Pick up sprint training

This increases the speed of work: it begins with walking, moving on to jogging, then striding and sprinting; ending up with walking again. The process is repeated as often as possible. This improves both aerobic and anaerobic systems and trains athletes to pick up speed quickly.

Other methods of aerobic training include cross training and circuit training.

Cross training

Many athletes derive benefit from cross training. This combines different forms of training; eg, cycling may be combined with swimming. The swimming will not improve cycling prowess, but it will maintain endurance qualities and allow recovery of cycling muscles.

Circuit training

Circuits are a selection of exercises, organised in sequence and performed in a specific order. They are designed to use a different muscle group at each station. They can be planned to improve aerobic endurance or to improve muscle strength or a combination of both; they are therefore useful for improving overall fitness.

Exercises can be interspersed with aerobic activity such as jogging, skipping, cycling, step-ups. This will increase the aerobic training effect. The exercises must be carefully selected depending on the objective; they should be planned so that muscle groups from different parts of the body are worked at consecutive stations – eg, exercising quadriceps, followed by the abdominals, and then biceps.

The load and number of repetitions and recovery period between each exercise will be organised according to the fitness level of the participants. The unfit will require a longer rest period than the fit; the rest period may vary from 20–60 seconds; for strength 30–60 seconds, and for endurance 0–10 seconds.

Circuits can be used for individual training or for groups. They provide variety which increases interest and motivation.

See Chapter 13 for **aerobic classes**.

Precautions

- Build up training gradually, do not exceed maximum heart rate (MHR). Remember that the unfit should begin at 60% MHR, working up to 80% or 90% as fitness develops.
- Do not exercise if there is any pain.
- Do not exercise if suffering from colds, fevers, flu, etc.

- Stop exercising if pain develops.
- Drink fluid after a training session or during long distance running to prevent dehydration.
- Wear well fitting, well cushioned, appropriate footwear.
- Wear loose absorbent clothing.

Endurance training effects

- The heart increases in size and volume.
- The efficiency of the heart improves: it pumps out a larger volume per beat (stroke volume) and therefore a larger quantity per minute (cardiac output).
- As fitness develops, the heart rate will be progressively lowered for the same workloads, indicating greater efficiency. The heart rests for a longer period, which reduces effort.
- The resting heart rate is considerably reduced; it may be down to 50 bpm. Highly trained athletes may have a heart rate as low as 40 bpm.
- There is an increase in the size and number of blood vessels to the heart and to skeletal muscle.
- There is an increase in capillary density to the heart and to skeletal muscle, therefore the delivery of oxygen and removal of waste will increase.
- Blood is shunted away from inactive organs to increase the supply to contracting muscles.
- There is an increase in the size and number of mitochondria in muscle cells, which enables oxygen to be utilised more efficiently and more energy to be produced.
- The muscles' capacity to store glycogen and glycolytic enzymes will increase.
- Rate and depth of respiration increases improving ventilation.
- Fats are utilised for energy production which reduces body fat.
- Bones are strengthened in response to stresses placed on them.
- Maximum oxygen uptake (VO_2 max) is raised with training. Average VO_2 max is around 40–45 ml/kg/min, but well trained endurance athletes may have a VO_2 max of 60–70 ml/kg/min.
- The anaerobic threshold is raised; aerobic metabolism is therefore used for longer periods, increasing the capacity to exercise without fatigue.

Muscle fitness

Muscle fitness relates to the *strength, bulk, power* and *endurance* of a muscle. Improvement is gained as muscles adapt in response to overload (applying the appropriate stress to gain improvement). The training programme must therefore be carefully designed to meet the set objectives and be specific to those muscles requiring improvement. The load, number of repetitions, number of sets, speed of contraction and the rest period can be varied to produce desired effects. The programme may be designed to improve any of the following:

1 *Muscle strength* is the ability to exert force against resistance. Strength will increase in response to a progressive overload over a period of time; ie, making the muscle contract against increasing resistance over a period of time. High resistance with low repetitions develops strength.

2 *Muscle bulk* relates to the size of a muscle. Working a muscle against overload will result in hypertrophy; ie, the cross-sectional measurement of the muscle increases. Muscle bulk and strength are interrelated: as size increases, so does strength. Weight lifting for bulking should include one or two lifts at maximal resistance.

3 *Muscle endurance* is a muscle's ability to contract repeatedly over a period of time against a force. Endurance will increase in response to lower resistance, but high, near maximum repetitions ie, making the muscle repeat a lift as many times as is possible with a low resistance. Low resistance but high repetition develops endurance.

4 *Muscle power and explosive power* is a combination of strength and speed. Plyometric training, where muscle contraction is performed following rapid stretch, is one method of improving power.

Methods of applying resistance

In general we think of weight training when we consider muscle fitness, but there are many other forms of resistance which may be effective and convenient to use. However, some of the methods are not measurable, which is a disadvantage as accurate progression cannot be recorded.

Muscles can be made to work against:

- Own body weight, eg, press ups (*calisthenics*) – not measurable.
- The resistance provided by a partner, eg, pushing or pulling against a partner – not measurable.
- Water may be used as resistance – not measurable.
- Rubber bands or elasticated straps etc. – not measurable.
- Free weights such as sand bags, weight boots, ankle and wrist weights, dumb bells and bar bells etc. – measurable.
- Springs and pulleys – measurable.
- Specialised equipment such as rowing machines, exercise bikes, multigyms, isokinetic machines, and the many other forms of resistance machines now on the market – measurable.

When using these machines or instructing others in their use, read the manufacturers' instructions carefully. Make sure that you are working the muscles you intended working, as the terminology used in the instructions is not always specific.

Muscle strength

Muscle strength is a basic requirement for all athletic and sport performance. It is often the most important factor in improving performance and achieving success at the highest level.

Muscle strength is the muscle's ability to apply force against resistance. A muscle's maximal strength is the greatest force it can develop against resistance. It is measured by the maximum weight that can be lifted in a single effort, which is known as one repetition maximum (1 RM). There are different methods of assessing this; a simple way is to use increasingly heavier weights until the maximum weight that can be lifted is reached.

Attempting repetitive lifts using this maximum weight is not recommended as it may result in muscle strain. One or two lifts at this weight may be performed if the aim is to increase bulk, but a partner should be to hand to assist, should the weight prove too heavy. Experienced lifters and body builders may include lifts of 100% RM in their routines.

As strength and bulk are interrelated, training for one will also improve the other. *Progressive overload* must be applied to increase strength. Progression is achieved by increasing

- the resistance (load)
- the repetitions
- the number of sets
- the number of training sessions.

The most important and effective of these is increasing the resistance (load).

Technique of strength training

Exercise schemes may be required for general body strengthening and/or for strengthening of specific muscles or groups. When strengthening muscles it is important to maintain a balance between both sides of the body and also between opposing muscles; ie, the agonists and antagonists. The programme must be designed to meet the requirements of the individual and must be appropriate to the level of fitness.

The principles of training apply as before. The overload must be gradually increased considering the three variables:

- Intensity: how much weight/resistance
- Duration: how many repetitions (lifts and sets)
- Frequency: how often

Strength may be improved by applying resistance to isometric work, isotonic work or isokinetic work.

Isometric strength training

This is static exercise: tension develops in the muscle but there is no change in length. Isometric contractions are useful in rehabilitation when pain may inhibit joint movement, and also in developing strength at specific weak points in the range.

For total strength, it is important to apply near maximal resistance at four to five different points (angles) throughout the range. Resistance can be applied by pushing or pulling against one's own or a partner's force, or by pushing against immovable objects such as the wall, table, floor, machines etc.

For example: double leg press to strengthen the quadriceps muscle:

- 5 contractions at the end of inner range
- 5 contractions at the beginning of middle range
- 5 contractions at the end of middle range
- 5 contractions at the end of outer range

Each contraction should be held for at least 5 seconds and repeated 5–10 times.

These exercises have the advantage that expensive equipment is not necessarily required. There are however disadvantages to isometric training.

DISADVANTAGES OF ISOMETRIC RESISTANCE

- It is difficult to ensure that the appropriate overload is applied, and to measure accurate progression.
- Strength is developed at the point where overload is applied and therefore is not developed through the entire range.
- There is no alternate contraction–relaxation of the muscle, therefore no pumping action to deliver blood. The maintained pressure on the capillary networks in the muscles prevents the delivery of nutrients and oxygen – fatigue will quickly develop.
- This type of exercise raises blood pressure; isometric work should NOT be performed by anyone with heart or blood pressure problems.

Isotonic strength training

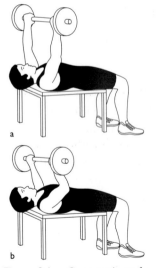

This is dynamic exercise: tension develops in the muscle, which may shorten or lengthen. Resistance may be applied to both concentric work (muscle shortening) and to eccentric work (muscle lengthening).

- As the muscle contracts to lift the weight, the resistance is applied to concentric work. This is referred to as the positive phase and is the more effective phase for increasing strength and bulk.
- Resistance is applied to eccentric work as the part is lowered back to the starting position. This is referred to as the negative phase.

For example, the lift up is concentric work for triceps, lowering back to starting position is eccentric work for triceps. The lowering, eccentric phase must take longer to perform than the concentric phase, to gain maximum effect. Although eccentric work produces muscle soreness, it is possible to use a heavier load for eccentric contraction. This technique is sometimes used by very experienced

Figure 8.1　*Concentric and eccentric phases of lifting (a) lifting, triceps concentric (b) lowering, triceps eccentric*

lifters as part of their routine. The technique involves using two assistants to lift a heavy load into position (slightly too heavy for the concentric phase), which is then lowered slowly by the lifter.

Isokinetic work

Special machines have been developed which automatically adapt the resistance so that speed and tension is maintained through the range, causing strength to develop evenly throughout the range. Research indicates that isokinetic work produces significant strength gains. It is effective in rehabilitation following injury, and in training for sports where strength is required throughout the range.

Uses of resistance training

1 To strengthen specific muscles required for sport, athletic performance, etc.
2 To improve speed and power.
3 To improve muscle endurance.
4 To strengthen specific muscles for improvement of posture.
5 To generally strengthen body muscles to improve body shape.
6 To increase lean body tissue and decrease body fat.
7 To rehabilitate muscles following injury.

Planning strengthening programmes

- Assess goals, establish to what end is improvement required. The goals should be realistic and achievable, and must be discussed and agreed with the client.
- Discuss and agree a time scale.
- Assess present level of strength – this will indicate the initial starting resistance and the repetitions. Record assessment data.
- Select the training method and the equipment.
- Plan the warm up.
- Plan the stretch routine.
- Plan the core conditioning phase.
- Plan cool down and include some stretch.
- Consider the rest or recovery time.
- Record the load, the number of repetitions and the number of sets.

■ Evaluate the progress at regular intervals, eg, every month.

General strength training

These schemes should include strengthening exercises for all the large muscle groups. General schemes may include exercises against gravity, against own body weight, against resistance from a partner or using weights such as dumb bells, poles, ankle and wrist weights, medicine balls, weight machines etc. They may be performed individually or as a class. Most aerobic exercise classes include some strengthening work.

A selection of exercises for specific muscle groups are listed at the end of this chapter.

Circuit training

Circuits can be used for general strengthening, similar to those used for aerobic conditioning, but each station (area) should provide a resisted exercise for one specific muscle or group. Six to ten stations are organised in a circle around the room and are carefully planned so that the client can progress easily from one to the other. It is important that the circuit is designed to use different muscles at each station, as this allows time for the muscles to recover from effort. Care must be taken to explain each movement before commencing the circuit, and each exercise should be practised with a light weight to ensure accuracy. The selected load and number of repetitions of each exercise will depend upon the level of fitness of the individual, and must be increased as strength develops.

EXAMPLE

Ten lifts at sub-maximal effort are performed at the first station, followed by a short 30–60 second rest (or longer, depending on fitness). Progress is made in this way around the circuit. The circuit is repeated two to three times in the same sequence, following a period of rest of two to three minutes or more, depending on fitness level. The training programme is repeated three to four times per week.

Circuits can be planned to offer weights, interspersed with aerobic activity such as jogging or cycling. This is an excellent way of improving strength and endurance.

Specific strength training

Here, progressive resistance is used to develop strength and bulk in specific muscles or muscle groups. There are many variations of overload techniques, and individuals respond better to some than others. The therapist must refer to specialist texts on resistance training in order to select the most suitable for the client. Although routines may vary, there are certain factors common to all.

Recording data

It is very important to record accurate details of the programme and progress. Measurements of bulk and strength taken at regular intervals under the same conditions will indicate progress. These measurements must be recorded before commencing the programme, and then every four weeks. Firstly:

- measure bulk with a tape measure placed around the widest point; always measure at the same point; record (see Chapter 14)
- measure strength by the maximum weight which can be lifted in a single lift (1 RM); record 1 RM

During each session, the following data must be recorded:

- the load (the weight that is lifted)
- the repetitions (the number of times the weight is lifted without a rest – it is usual to select 6–10 lifts)
- the number of sets performed. Select 1–5 sets and allow 1 minute rest period between each set. These are recorded as follows:
    10 kg × 8 reps × 3 sets
  As strength develops, the weight or number of sets is increased.

For improving strength, 'heavy load low repetitions' is the format: the weight lifted should be at least two thirds of the maximum possible weight – over 66% of 1 RM. Beginners should practise initially with low weights until they have perfected the technique.

It is possible to vary the routines; the following are examples of effective but simple systems.

EXAMPLE I

Establish 1 RM and calculate 80% of this, which will be the starting weight. If 1 RM = 25 kg, the weight will be 20 kg.

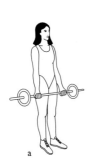
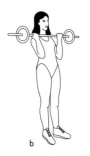

Figure 8.2 *Weight lift for biceps strength*

This would be lifted 6–8 times and recorded as:

20 kg × 8 × 1
20 kg × 8 × 2
20 kg × 8 × 3

EXAMPLE 2

Establish 10 RM (the weight that can be lifted 10 times). The first set of 10 lifts is performed with 50% of this weight, the second set with 75% and the third set with 100%. If 10 RM was 20 kg, this would be recorded as:

10 kg × 10 × 1
15 kg × 10 × 2
20 kg × 10 × 3

The weight is increased as strength develops. The repetitions and sets may also be increased, but increasing the weight is the most essential.

Allow 48 hours between training sessions to ensure adequate recovery.

The pyramid method

The pyramid method is effective for strength, bulk and endurance. As the weight increases, the repetitions decrease; if the weight decreases, the repetitions increase. The maximum weight that can be lifted twice is assessed (ie, 2 RM), and the pyramid is constructed from that starting point. A one-sided regime is sometimes used, working up to maximum weight and then resting for 1–2 minutes.

EXAMPLE

If 2 RM is 5 kg:

- 5 repetitions at 2 kg
- 4 repetitions at 3 kg
- 3 repetitions at 4 kg
- 2 repetitions at 5 kg
- 3 repetitions at 4 kg
- 4 repetitions at 3 kg
- 5 repetitions at 2 kg.

Precautions to be observed during strength training

- Set realistic objectives.
- Select weights appropriate to strength level.
- Check weights for safety.

- Start with an easy programme with light weights and few lifts.
- Perform warm up.
- Choose a correct stable starting position.
- Secure the weights so that they cannot move or slide.
- Keep good body alignment.
- Perform the lift carefully and slowly for maximum effect with a heavy weight (momentum plays a part in fast movement – it is less effective and can result in trauma). Fast movement with low weight for endurance is safer.
- The rest between each lift should be minimal 1–2 seconds. The rest between each set should be 1–2 minutes to allow for recovery.
- Increase number of lifts up to 30 and then increase the weight when 2–3 extra lifts can be performed.
- Do not hold the breath when lifting, as this can cause an increase in blood pressure and increases the load on the heart. Holding the breath can also increase intra-abdominal pressure which can cause hernia. Keep mouth open and breathe regularly.
- Exhale as you lift, inhale as you lower.
- Work different muscle groups. Change the exercises so that different muscles are stressed. Allow recovery time.
- Maintain a balance between agonist and antagonist.
- Replace weights and all apparatus neatly and safely.

Effects of strength training

The physiological effects of muscle strengthening are:

- The recruitment of more motor units, which increases the strength of the contraction.
- A faster neuro-muscular response, which increases the speed of contraction.
- An increase in the size and number of myofibrils, which increases strength and bulk. Recent research indicates that in some instances there may be an increase in the number of muscle fibres.
- An increase in contractile proteins myosine and actine.
- An increase in ATP, PC, enzymes and glycogen stores.
- An increase in blood flow to the muscles due to dilation (although there is no increase in the number of blood vessels or capillary networks as with endurance training).
- An increase in the mineral content of bones.
- An increase in strength of tendons and ligaments.

On average, the absolute strength in males is greater than in females. This is due to body composition and the fact that males bulk more readily than females. Research indicates that this is due to the increased presence of the male hormone testosterone, which is necessary for the synthesis of actin and myosin. However, females will develop strength in response to progressive weight training.

Muscles do not respond equally to programmes of equal intensity. The average rate of strength gain is around 5% per week, but some muscles gain only 1%, while gains of 100% have been recorded. Gains are greatest in the more active, fitter muscles and fast twitch fibres are more responsive to resistance training than slow twitch fibres. Improvement is greatest at the beginning of a strength training programme, levelling out as the programme continues.

Dangers of strength training

- Muscle strain and even rupture of fibres if too much overload is applied.
- Muscle fatigue and soreness if repetitions are too high and rest periods are too short.
- Trauma – if weights are not properly secure they may fall and cause damage.
- Damage to the moving joints and their connective tissue components if the positioning of the join is incorrect or if the lifts are casually performed.
- Overstress of other joints through poor posture and poor technique.

Muscle endurance

This is the ability of the muscles to perform continuously over a period of time (ie, performing repeated contractions). Muscle endurance is dependent upon:

- an adequate supply of oxygen and nutrients delivered by the circulating blood
- the efficiency of muscle cells in utilising these substances to produce energy
- the efficient removal of waste products from the muscle.

The main difference between training for endurance as opposed to strength is that *lighter weights are used and repetitions are increased.* For endurance, the weight is usually kept below 66% of maximum weight, around 40–60% of 1 RM and repeated 20–30 times per set for up to three sets. Training must be repeated 3–5 times per week.

Speed can also be improved using high speed contractions with low resistance.

Endurance training effects

- Increase in number and size of blood vessels to the muscles.
- Increase in the number of capillary networks supplying the muscles.
- Increase in mitochondria in muscle cells.
- Increase in oxidative enzymes which extract oxygen from the blood. Therefore the aerobic capacity of the muscles is improved.
- Increase in glycogen stores used for energy.

Plyometrics

Explosive power will improve using *plyometrics.* These are jumping, leaping, hopping movements, where the prime mover is stretched before contraction. The speed of the stretch is an important factor. When a muscle is stretched, the stretch receptors within the muscle are stimulated. This increases the strength of the following contraction. The longer and faster the stretch, the greater the following concentric contraction.

There is a danger of damaging joints and producing micro-tears in muscle fibres when performing these exercises. They must only be performed under expert tuition, by the very fit and only after adequate warm up.

Suggested routines for muscle fitness

The wide range of values for weight, reps, sets and rest allow for variations in fitness levels. Beginners will start well below or at the low end and progress gradually; intermediate lifters will work in the middle ranges and advanced lifters in the upper ranges.

Table 8.1   Summary of suggested routines

	IRM	Reps	Sets	Pace	Rest between sets or lifts
Strength	80–95%	2–6	3–5	medium	1–4 minutes between sets
Power	80–90%	2–6	3–5	fast	1–2 minutes between sets
Bulk	70–90%	6–12	3–10	slow	long rest between sets as required
Endurance	40–60%	15–30	15–30	fast	little or no rest between lifts

Note: experienced body builders training for bulk may include 1–2 lifts at 100% 1 RM

Following training sessions, the muscles must be given an adequate amount of time to recover. At least 48 hours is recommended, which will allow for training every other day providing there is no injury.

It must be remembered that training should be consistent and regular. If training ceases, the effects of training will regress and fitness levels will return to pre-training levels. Strength regresses more quickly than skill. The effects of training over a long period, will remain for a longer period after training stops. The effects of short duration training, regress more quickly.

Strengthening exercises

The following exercises are designed to gradually increase in intensity and increase muscle strength from a very basic level. They could be selected for use in rehabilitation, correction of posture, to meet the needs of specific sports or in general activity classes.

Calf strengthening: Gastrocnemius and Soleus, Plantar flexors

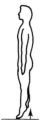

STARTING POSITION	EXERCISE
Standing	Lift up onto toes and down.
Standing on one leg	Lift up onto toes and down. Repeat with other leg.
Standing	Step onto a step then lift onto toes. Repeat other leg.

When these three exercises become too easy and the client can perform 20–30 without difficulty, weights can be used to increase the effort. Hold equal weights in each hand, begin with 1 kg and increase gradually as muscle strength improves.

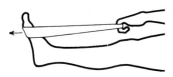

Long sitting with resistance rubber belt around the feet and pull with hands	Push both feet against the belt then push alternate feet against the belt. or Use multigym and plantar flex against the resistance.

The following activities will also improve strength as well as mobility of the foot and ankle.
Walking: push off onto toes
Jumping: pushing from toes
Hop on one foot and then the other
Skip on the toes
Sprint from one wall to another
Run or jog on a flat surface
Run or jog up a hill
Jump across a bench, bunny jumps or straight
Work on a wobble board

Quadriceps strengthening: Rectus femoris, vastus medialis, vastus lateralis, vastus intermedius: Knee extensors

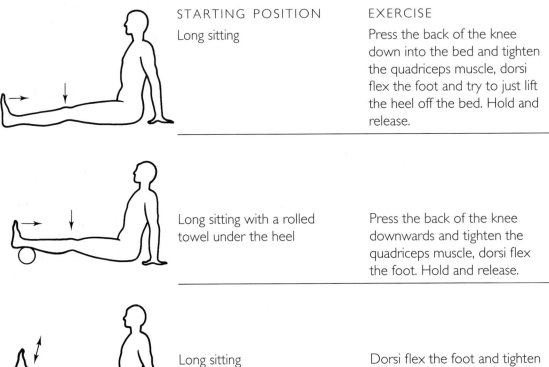

STARTING POSITION	EXERCISE
Long sitting	Press the back of the knee down into the bed and tighten the quadriceps muscle, dorsi flex the foot and try to just lift the heel off the bed. Hold and release.
Long sitting with a rolled towel under the heel	Press the back of the knee downwards and tighten the quadriceps muscle, dorsi flex the foot. Hold and release.
Long sitting	Dorsi flex the foot and tighten the knee. Raise the leg just off the bed, keeping the knee tight and straight.

If the knee bends slightly, it indicates that the muscle is weak and that the above exercises must be continued until the leg can be lifted without any give.

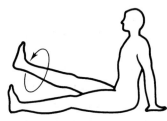

Long sitting	Dorsi flex the foot and tighten the knee, then lift the leg and circle slowly around.
Long sitting	Dorsi flex the foot and tighten the knee, lift the leg and lower almost to the bed, then lift again several times.

Long sitting	Dorsi flex the foot and tighten the knee, lift the leg and swing out sideways and back, repeat several times.
Long sitting with tightly rolled towel behind knee under thigh	Dorsi flex the foot and lift the lower leg to straighten the knee, then lower.

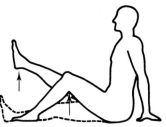

Crook sitting	Straighten alternate legs upwards to straighten knee.
Long sitting – place a weight across the ankle, begin with a weight that can just be lifted with a straight knee	Dorsi flex the foot, clear the heel off the ground as the knee is tightened. Then lift the leg and weight off the bed. Hold and lower. (Do not lift too high – 24 cms or so.)

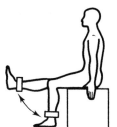

Long sitting with rolled towel behind the knee, weight over ankle as above	Press the back of the knee into the towel and straighten the knee. Hold and release.
High sitting on a high chair or on the edge of a couch, feet must be off the floor and knee at 90°. Weight strapped to ankle as above.	Slowly lift the weight until the knee is straight. Keep the thigh in contact with the couch. Hold and lower slowly back to 90° bend. Repeat 10 times, then rest for 1 minute. Repeat again until weight is lifted 30 times. Then increase weight.

Again, if the knee cannot fully straighten the weight is too great. Repeat with a lower weight.

This exercise can be performed with an elasticated band or spring attached behind the chair, level with the ankle; the leg then pulls against it. Use leg press machine if available. Before using weights to improve strength, read the notes on weight training, page 128.

Wing standing	Bend the knees and lower the body slowly bending to just above a right angle. Keep the back straight. Push up straight and lock knees by pulling patella upwards. (*Caution:* do not take buttocks below knee)

This can be progressed by holding a weight in the arms or placing them over the shoulders. A fit person could perform this with one leg at a time.

Using a multigym or sliding sprung board or rowing machine.	Bend knees fully. Then push out to straighten and tighten the knees, hold and bend slowly. Keep the back straight.
Stand in front of a bench or stairs	Step up a straighten knee fully, then down. Do ten or more per leg.
Climb the stairs two at a time	

Cycling: make sure that the leg can straighten on each downward movement of the pedal. Increase the resistance as necessary on exercise bikes or cycle up hill on an ordinary bicycle.

Hamstring strengthening: Biceps femoris, semimenbranosus, semitendinosus. Knee flexors and hip extensors

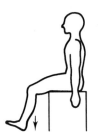

STARTING POSITION	EXERCISE
High sitting, heel resting on floor	Press alternate heels into the floor.

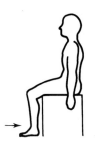

High sitting with heels against the chair legs	Press the back of the heel alternately into the chair legs. Progress by sitting forward so that the knee is bent to a greater angle.

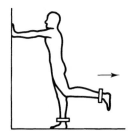

Standing	Bend alternate knees to a right angle and extend the hip (push it backwards).
Standing with weight around ankles	Bend alternate knees to a right angle and extend hip. Progress by extending with a straight leg.

Prone lying	Cross legs at the ankles, bend the underneath leg and resist with the top leg.
Prone lying with weights around ankle	Bend alternate knees to right angle and lift leg upwards from the hip.
Prone lying, bend knees with elastic strap or spring tied to ankle and behind at ankle level, or use multigym.	Bend the knee to a right angle against the resistance.

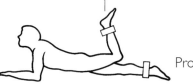

Hip Extensor strengthening: hamstrings and Gluteus maximus

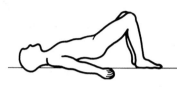

STARTING POSITION	EXERCISE
Supine lying or high sitting	Tighten buttocks then release.
Supine lying	Tighten buttocks and lift slightly off the floor.
Crook lying	Lift buttocks off the floor.
Standing	Swing alternate legs forwards and backwards and lower slowly.
Stride standing	Slide arms down the legs, bend trunk forwards and return to upright.

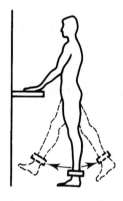

Standing with weights on ankles	Swing alternate legs backwards and lower slowly.

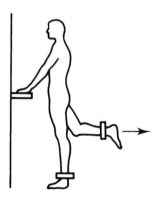

Standing with weights on ankles	Bend knee to right angles and press leg with short movements backwards.
High sitting	Stand up and sit down slowly.

	High sitting	Press thighs downwards into seat and rotate outwards.
	Prone lying – bend knees	Lift alternate legs off the floor. (*Caution:* keep hips against floor) Ankle weights can be used for progression.
	Prone lying	Lift both legs off the floor. (*Caution:* keep hips against floor)
	Prone kneeling	Lift leg backwards and upwards (ankle weights can be used for progression).
	Prone lying with weights around ankle	Lift alternate legs off the floor.
	Stoop standing with trunk supported on the bed	Raise alternate legs backwards and upwards. Keep knee straight and hips on the bed. Ankle weights can be used for progression.
	Prone lying on couch with one leg over the edge	Lift this leg backwards and upwards. Repeat with other leg. Repeat with weights around ankles.

Abductor strengthening: Glutus medius, gluteus minimus and tensor fascia lata. Hip abductors and medial rotators

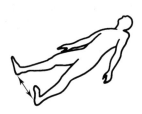

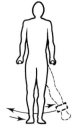

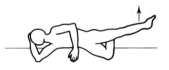

STARTING POSITION	EXERCISE
Supine lying	Part legs and close them.
Supine lying	Lift alternate legs slightly, move out to side and return.
High sitting or lying with feet inside the legs of a chair	Push both legs outwards against legs of the chair, hold then release.
As above	Use partner and push against her legs.
Support standing	Keep the back straight and swing alternate legs slowly out sideways and back across other leg. Occasionally hold the leg in abduction.
Support standing with weights on ankles	As above, swing alternate legs slowly out sideways and back across other leg. Hold in abduction.
Side lying, bend underneath leg for balance.	Lift upper leg, hold and lower. Keep the hip pushed forward throughout. Progress using weights.

Note: When this exercise is performed correctly, only 35–40° of abduction is possible due to the structure of the joint. Individuals are seen to gain greater range by rolling the hip backward but this brings the hip flexors into play and therefore is not working the abductors.

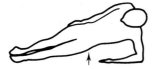

Side lying with weight on elbow	Push pelvis upwards to arch away from the floor.

Adductor strengthening: Adductor magnus adductor longus, adductor brevis, pectineus and gracilis. Hip adductors and lateral rotators

STARTING POSITION	EXERCISE
Supine lying	Part legs and close them.
Supine lying	Lift alternate legs slightly, move out to the side and back across the other leg.
Supine lying	Bend knees onto chest and then straighten legs into the air, keep at 90°. Scissor legs open and across.
High sitting or lying with feet outside the legs of a chair	Push both legs inwards against the legs of the chair, hold then release.
As above	Use a partner and push against her legs.
Crook lying	Part knees then close them. Repeat with hands on inside of knees pushing against the movement.
Crook lying	Place pillow or firm sponge between the knees and press knees together.
Support standing	Keep the back straight, swing alternate legs out slowly sideways and return across other leg, hold and release.

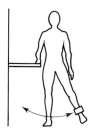

Support standing with weights on ankles

As above, swing alternate legs out slowly sideways and return slowly across other leg, hold and release.

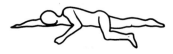

Side lying, bend upper leg place in front

Raise under leg upwards, hold and release.
Progress using heavier weights.

Abdominal strengthening: Rectus abdominus, the external oblique, internal oblique, transversus abdominus. Trunk flexors, side flexors and rotators

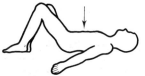

STARTING POSITION	EXERCISE
Crook lying	Press the small of the back into the floor, tilt pelvis backwards, pull stomach in. Hold and release.
Crook lying	Press the small of the back into the floor. Tuck the head down onto the chest, then raise head and shoulders to look at the knees. Hold and release.
Crook lying	Bring both knees up to form a right angle at hip and knee. Reach up towards ceiling with alternate knees.
Crook lying arms at side	Curl up to knees. (*Caution:* return slowly from base of spine upwards)
Crook lying, arms across chest	Curl up to knees.

Crook lying, hands on shoulders	Curl up to knees.

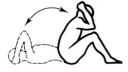

Crook lying, hands on ears (not behind the neck as the pull of the hands can damage the neck)	Curl up towards knees.
Crook lying, arms stretched above head (keep arms back, do not swing forward)	Curl up towards knees. (*Caution:* only for those with strong abdominals)
Crook lying, holding weight – medicine ball on chest	Curl up towards knees. (*Caution: only for those with strong abdominals*)
Crook lying, holding weight – medicine ball above head	Curl up towards knees. (*Caution: only for those with strong abdominals*)

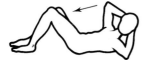

Crook lying, hands on shoulders	Twist to touch right elbow towards left knee, return and repeat with opposite side.
Reach, crook lying	Curl up and take both arms to outside of opposite leg, return and repeat on either side.
Crook lying	Bend knees onto chest and then stretch legs towards ceiling. Reach upwards to ceiling.
Crook lying	Bend knees onto chest and then stretch legs towards ceiling. Keep feet together and make small circles in the air.

Back strengthening: Erector spinae, and quadratus lumborum. Back extensors and side flexors

STARTING POSITION	EXERCISE
Prone lying	Lift alternate legs up and lower.
Prone lying arms outstretched	Lift alternate arms up and lower.
Prone lying arms outstretched	Stretch left arm and right leg along the floor, then lift slightly and release, repeat with other arm and leg.
Prone lying arms to sides	Keep the chin in (to the chest) and lift the head and shoulders then lower slowly.
Prone lying hands clasped behind back	Keep chin in elbows straight, lift the head and shoulders then lower slowly.
Prone lying arms outstretched	Keep chin in, lift arms, head and shoulders then lower slowly. This may be progressed holding weight in the hands.
Prone lying arms to side with the head and shoulders over the edge of the bed (fix the feet)	Lift the head and shoulders as high as possible then slowly lower.
As above with hands on shoulders	Lift the arms, head and shoulders as high as possible then slowly lower.

These exercises should not be undertaken by anyone with back problems or pain.

Trapezius and rhomboids strengthening: Retractors of the shoulder girdle

STARTING POSITION	EXERCISE
Stride standing	Circle the shoulders backwards alternately and then together.
Stride standing	Pull the shoulders down and backwards.
Across bend stride standing	Pull elbows backwards, release, straighten arms and pull backwards.

This exercise commonly called 'pull pull fling' should be done slowly and deliberately, as too fast a movement activates the stretch reflex within the muscle and may result in microtears of myofibrils (see Chapter 9).

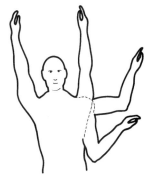

Standing heels 10 cm approximately away from wall	Flatten the back against the wall, stretch arms above the head, palms facing forward. Keep the back against the wall and slide the arms down along the wall bending the elbows. Slide the arms up and down the wall.
High sitting, hands on thighs	Bend forward chest to thighs. Raise the trunk inch by inch pushing into the back of the chair.

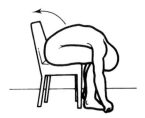

High sitting	Bend forward as above, raise trunk against the resistance of a therapist applying force behind the shoulders.
Prone lying	Keep the chin in, raise head and shoulders off the floor, hold and release, lower slowly.

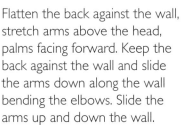

Prone lying hands clasped behind back	Chin in, pull shoulders back and lift head and shoulders off the floor, hold and lower slowly.
Prone lying hands on shoulders	Chin in, pull shoulders back and lift head and shoulders off the floor, hold and lower slowly.
Yard prone lying	Chin in, lift arms backwards and raise head and shoulders off the floor.

Serratus anterior and triceps strengthening: Positioning of scapula during movements of the arm and holding the scapula against the chest wall. The same exercises are used for the extensor of the elbow triceps

STARTING POSITION	EXERCISE
Across bend stride standing	Pull elbows back and straighten arms out to side slowly and deliberately.
Bend stride standing	Punch the air, a pillow, punch bag or therapist's hands.
Bend stride standing	Push forwards against the resistance of the therapist, first with both hands, then alternately.
Bend stride standing	Straighten arms up above head alternately and then together.
Stride standing or high sitting	Lean body forwards, straighten arms and stretch backwards (hand weights can be used for progression).
Stride standing arms bend, hands on wall	Push the body away from the wall by straightening the elbows.
Prone kneeling	Bend and straighten the elbows.

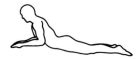

Prone lying	Bend and straighten the elbows lifting upper trunk (half press up).
Prone lying	Press up.

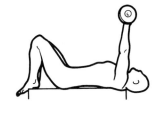

Crook lying holding weights in hands at shoulder level	Push weights vertically upwards and lower, first alternately then together. Progress by increasing the weights.

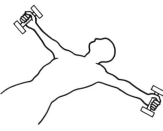

Yard crook lying	Hold weights, raise arms from side to ceiling. Progress by increasing the weights.

These exercises should not be performed by a client with round shoulders as they strengthen the pectoral muscles.

Speed

Speed is the distance moved in a specific time:

$$\text{Speed} = \frac{\text{distance moved}}{\text{time taken}}$$

Speed is required in many athletic and sporting activities. It is dependent on the length of the stride and frequency of the stride; increasing one or both of these factors will increase running speed. These factors will depend on the length of the limbs and the power of muscle contraction, and also on co-ordination and timing. Speed is required in the lower limbs for sprinting, in the upper limbs for throwing or fast bowling, and in both for certain sports such as basketball. Speed is therefore related to many factors such as muscle strength, flexibility, reaction time and leverage. Factors which can adversely affect speed include the build up of lactic acid, friction, resistance force and mass.

Factors which positively affect speed

Muscle strength

This is required to produce the force necessary for acceleration. The greater the force applied by the muscles, the greater the acceleration and speed; the greater the force generated by the muscles, the higher the energy expenditure.

In sprinting, the push off muscles of the propelling leg will drive the body forward. The greater the strength of these muscles, the greater the driving force. These muscles are gastrocnemius and soleus in the calf, the quadriceps on the front of the thigh and gluteus maximus in the buttock. Strengthening exercises for these muscles should form part of the training regime to increase running speed.

For throwing speed, strengthening exercises to serratus anterior, pectoralis major, anterior deltoid, triceps, wrist and finger extensors are required.

Flexibility

Flexibility is required to provide maximum range of movement at joints. This will allow for longer strides, and long fast strides will increase speed. Increased flexibility of the ankle, knee and hip will increase running speed; increased flexibility of the shoulder, elbow and wrist will increase the propulsion force when throwing. Flexibility exercises should be included in training programmes.

Reaction time

This is the ability to react quickly to a stimulus which is vital in running and in most sports. Muscles must be able to contract instantly in response to a stimulus such as a starting gun, or the hit of a service ball. Instant reactions to stimuli will improve speed. Reaction time can be improved by repetitive practice of the required action, maximising body position and nervous response. Exercises should be practised where quick response is required; eg, catching objects, striking a ball, pushing off the starting block.

Leverage

Leverage has an effect on speed, and body activities involve the movement of many levers. As explained in Chapter 5, the levers of the human body are mainly of the third order. These are designed for speed and range of movement. The longer the lever (longer bones), the greater range and speed, providing the force (muscle strength) is great enough.

Factors which adversely affect speed

Lactic acid

The build up of lactic acid affects speed because it has an inhibitory effect on muscle contraction. A burst of fast activity initially uses stored ATP and PC, but this is soon used up. Fast energy is then obtained from anaerobic partial breakdown of glycogen to pyruvic acid and lactic acid. This build up of lactic acid increases pressure within the muscle, restricts blood flow and the delivery of oxygen. This inhibits muscle contraction, which in turn reduces speed. Therefore athletes must train to increase their aerobic capacity and to run close to VO_2 max.

With use of aerobic metabolism for a longer period, there will be little or no lactic acid and little impairment of muscle action. This form of training will consist initially of short bursts of intense activity for 30–60 seconds, and then rests of the same duration. The time is then progressively increased. These activities may include shuttle running or a circuit of set exercises, interspersed with running.

Resistance

Speed will be affected by any form of resistance such as body weight or running against a wind. The greater the resistance, the slower the speed, but as muscle strength increases, the retarding effect will decrease.

Friction forces

These will also affect speed. The friction between the foot and the ground should be just enough to prevent slipping, but not great enough to retard movement.

Impact forces

As speed will be affected by reaction forces back from the ground, it is easier to run on hard surfaces than on soft surfaces (the reaction force is greater from hard surfaces). Speed will increase for the same effort.

Training for speed

This involves different forms of running; eg, beginning with jogging, moving on to running and finishing with maximum-speed sprinting, or maximum-speed running interspersed with walking or jogging.

Specific training which involves running at maximum speed for a set distance must also be included. This could be 50 metre sprints run at maximum speed, a set number of times.

Questions

1   Explain briefly what is meant by cardio-respiratory fitness.
2   At what level of intensity should an individual exercise in order to improve cardio-respiratory endurance?
3   Explain briefly how you would calculate an individual's maximum heart rate.
4   At what percentage of maximum heart rate should a beginner exercise?
5   List ten important effects of endurance training.
6   Define the following terms
   A Muscle strength
   B Muscle endurance

7   Explain what is meant by the term 'One repetition maximum'.
8   List four disadvantages of isometric strength training.
9   Explain briefly how you would construct a circuit for strengthening the large muscle groups of the legs and arms. Name the muscles and explain the selected exercise.
10 List six effects of muscle strength training.
11 Explain the principal difference between training for muscle strength and muscle endurance.

CHAPTER 9

Flexibility and Suppleness

This refers to the range of movement possible at a joint or group of joints. A joint will move through a range of movement from one point to another; eg, from full flexion to full extension, or other points in between (see page 105).

Flexibility is specific to each joint, which must be considered separately. However, most activities (such as throwing a ball) will require flexibility at more than one joint, therefore the movement at each one must be considered. Flexibility is vital to the athlete and sportsperson as it contributes to

■ efficient technique
■ improved performance
■ prevention of injury

It can be increased through regular flexibility training and stretch exercises. These should be included after warm up and cool down in all training programmes.

Factors which affect flexibility

■ Joint structure
■ Age
■ Training
■ Sex
■ Body temperature
■ Strength training.

Joint structure

This is the main factor influencing flexibility. It includes:

■ the shape and contour of the articulating surfaces (the tighter the fit, the more limited the range)
■ the tension of the connective tissue components (the capsule and supporting ligaments)

■ the tension of the muscles and tendons acting on and surrounding the joint, which is governed by the stretch reflex. Where there is muscle imbalance, flexibility will be limited by the tight muscles.

Age

Ageing generally reduces flexibility, but training and activity will influence the degree of loss. Young children are very flexible, and depending on the level of activity, this flexibility continues to increase up to adolescence around 15 years. After the age of 15 years there is a natural decrease in flexibility. The rate of decrease will depend upon the activities, exercise and training practised by the individual; flexibility will decrease more slowly in those individuals who exercise regularly. Research indicates that flexibility can be increased for all age groups if appropriate exercises are undertaken, but the rate of increase will be greater in the younger age groups and will decline with age.

Training

Training and the selection of appropriate exercise will increase flexibility for all age groups. Those individuals such as gymnasts and ballet dancers who have continued with uninterrupted training programmes, will have greater flexibility than the untrained.

Sex

It has been suggested that females are more flexible than males, although the evidence is inconclusive. Females on the whole have lighter and smaller bones which may influence greater flexibility. In the main they have a shorter leg length and lower centre of gravity, making certain movements easier. They are also designed for flexibility of the pelvic region to facilitate child birth.

Body temperature

Elevation of body temperature increases flexibility. Therefore warm up exercises must be performed before flexibility training. Pre-heating with hot packs, heat lamps, hot baths or showers, diathermy or massage will increase the effect. The heat reduces viscosity and relaxes tissues such as the capsule and ligaments, which in turn offer less resistance to movement. Heat also increases the extensibility of muscle fibres and the tendons surrounding the joint, therefore flexibility increases.

Strength training

Certain strength training routines can limit joint flexibility if the joint is always moved through a limited range. Strength training must be planned to include full range movements and eccentric work.

Methods of maintaining and increasing flexibility

Flexibility can be *maintained* by the regular practice of full range and outer range movements; ie, exercises where the joint or joints are taken through to full stretch. However, flexibility can only be *increased* by overstretching. In the same way as we overload a muscle in order to increase strength, we must overstretch in order to increase flexibility. The body continually adapts to increasing demand placed upon it, therefore moving a joint beyond its existing range and stretching the surrounding tissues will result in increased range as the tissues become more extensible.

Flexibility programmes regularly practised, will increase the range of movement at the selected joints. Stretch exercises practised after warm up will enhance performance and reduce the risk of injury. They should also be performed during cool down to reduce muscle soreness and stiffness. Stretching exercises can also be used as a complete programme designed to progressively increase the range in joints throughout the body. This type of slow stretch programme allows time for thought and meditation, and as in yoga, pursues harmony of body, mind and spirit.

There are various methods of stretching, including:

- ballistic
- dynamic
- static
- proprioceptive neuromuscular facilitation (PNF).

Ballistic stretching

This type of stretching involves fast jerky movements where the increased momentum of the bounce is used to increase movement at the end of the range (eg, bouncing to touch toes).

Note: Ballistics are not generally recommended and should be avoided in class work. The arguments against their use are physiologically sound:

- A quick or rapid stretch does not allow sufficient time for the tissues to adapt, resulting in strain.
- A sudden jerk applied to a muscle will initiate the stretch reflex which results in rapid contraction to resist the stretch. This is a protective reflex mechanism, as increased muscle tension will prevent over-stretching of the muscle. Further pulling against this tension may result in microscopic tears of the myofibrils. Healing will occur with formation of non elastic fibrous tissue, which will impair the function of the muscle.
- A quick stretch does not allow for neurological adaptation. Research has shown that the tension generated in a muscle by fast stretch is far greater than that generated by slow stretch. Therefore the tensile resistance to fast stretch is much greater.
- Bouncing movements are not easy to control. Therefore the positioning of joints and direction of movement may not be correct, increasing the likelihood of injury.

Despite all these reasons against ballistics, some people still use them for specific training. Gymnasts and dancers may practise them prior to specific actions or routines, but generally they should be avoided.

Dynamic stretching

These are movements where a muscle or group of muscles are worked gradually through their range (some texts group these movements as ballistic). Beginning with short range movements, the actions move progressively through to maximum full range. Dynamic flexibility is required by ball kickers in rugby and soccer, and in shot putters and javelin throwers; eg, gradual stretching of the hamstrings before kicking, by performing small range flexion/extension movements of the knee, building up to full range movement, will ensure that the action of the muscles used in kicking the ball is not hampered by tight hamstrings.

Static stretching

This form of stretching is the most effective and most commonly used. Movements are performed which take a muscle slowly and deliberately to the end of the range. The position is held and further stretch applied. During the holding time, the muscle adapts to the stretch. The stretch reflex is inhibited, there is a slow decrease in muscle tension and the muscle relaxes. This allows an increase in muscle length and in range of joint movement.

Research has shown that low force, long duration stretching at a raised temperature will result in permanent lengthening of muscles and connective tissue components.

Static stretching is safer and more effective than ballistic stretching as the tissues have time to relax. Maximum stretch is achieved when a muscle is fully relaxed and connective tissue fully stretched. The stretch reflex is inhibited, so that there is no risk of tearing, muscle soreness and damage. Movements are slower, more controlled and more functionally accurate, so there is less risk of injury. Static stretching requires less energy consumption than ballistics.

Static stretching may be classified into active or passive stretching:

- Active stretching refers to stretching alone, without external aid.
- Active assisted stretching refers to a stretch performed alone until a limit is reached, and then a partner applies pressure to help gain further stretch.

- Passive stretching refers to a stretch by an external force, such as traction or force by a partner, while the individual remains inactive.

All static stretching must be controlled and performed with care. Effective communication and total confidence must exist between partners performing active-assisted and passive stretching. These should only be practised by competent, well trained individuals.

Technique of static stretching

- Select a suitable venue which is warm and well ventilated. Ensure that there is sufficient space to perform all movements.
- Wear warm clothing to maintain and increase body temperature.
- Check that the floor surface is clean, smooth and non-slip.
- Do not stretch if any of the following contra-indications are present:
  Hyper mobility, strains or sprains, inflammation of joints, pain in joints, fevers, heart problems, high/low blood pressure, after a heavy meal.
- Identify the goals (where is flexibility required). Always warm up with a set of exercises designed to work the large muscle groups. The warm up should increase muscle temperature, reduce viscosity, decrease muscle tension, promote relaxation and will make tissues more extensible.
- Set the mind into a tranquil and relaxed state.
- Isolate the muscle or group for stretching and place the joint in the correct position. Stretch slowly and evenly, feel the pull *in the belly* of the muscle and not at the tendon ends. There should be a feeling of mild discomfort, but not pain. Hold the stretch for 6–10 seconds to begin, increasing to 20–30 seconds over time. As the tension decreases, stretch a little further – do not jerk or bounce at the end of movement. Let pain be the guide. If pain increases, relax; if muscle begins to quiver, relax; if muscle tension increases, relax. Move slowly out of the stretch.
- Repeat stretch five times at the beginning of a programme, eventually working up to 10–15.
- Exhale and relax as you move into the stretch.
- Stretching programmes should be performed once or twice a day if possible, if rapid improvement is required.

Proprioceptive Neuromuscular Facilitation (PNF)

There are many PNF techniques which are an excellent way of increasing range of movement, but they require an in-depth knowledge of neurophysiology and are not within the scope of this book. However, one of the techniques is straightforward and useful, especially following recovery from injury. (It should however only be practised by competent, well trained individuals.)

Alternate contract relax

An increased range is achieved in the following way:

- move a muscle to its point of slight stretch ie, at the end of joint movement
- perform an isometric contraction of that muscle against resistance
- hold
- follow with relaxation and further joint movement which will now be possible.

EXAMPLES

1 In prone lying (face down), lift one leg to stretch the hip flexors. Ask a friend to support the leg and to resist an isometric contraction (ie, you push down against her hand, but she must not allow movement). Relax, then lift the leg higher as the hip flexors allow greater range of movement.
2 Tilt the head to the left to stretch the right sterno-cleido-mastoid. Now place the hand against the right side of the face. Contract the muscle statically against the hand resistance, hold, and relax. The head will now move further to the left.

Effects of stretch training

- Increased range of movement at joints.
- Increased flexibility of supporting structures.
- Increased elasticity and length of muscles.
- Reduced tension and increased relaxation in muscles.
- Increased circulation to muscles.
- Improved balance and co-ordination between muscle groups.

- Improved posture.
- Improved mechanical efficiency therefore improved speed and skill.
- Improved technique and performance, relaxation of the antagonistic muscles allows the agonist to maximise performance.
- If performed after exercise and eccentric work, it reduces muscle soreness.

Stretching exercises

Stretching for foot

STARTING POSITION	EXERCISE
Sitting legs crossed at knee	Gently and evenly pull toes upwards and then the foot. Hold and relax.
Sitting legs crossed at knee	Gently and evenly push foot downwards and then toes. Hold and relax.
Heel sitting	With barefeet, sit back on heels and feel the pull on the top of the foot. Hold and relax. (*Caution:* not to be performed by anyone with knee problems.)
Standing	Place toes vertically against a step and rock forwards and raise heels off the ground.

Calf stretching: Gastrocnemius and Soleus

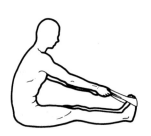

STARTING POSITION	EXERCISE
Long sitting, back against wall	Keep the knees straight and strongly dorsi flex the feet (do not invert or evert). Hold to 10 and release. (A strap can be used around the balls of the feet and pulled towards the body for additional stretch.)

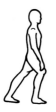	Walk standing, place one foot directly in front of the other	Keep back heel firmly on the ground, bend the front knee gently until you feel a pull in the calf of the hind leg. Hold for 10 then slowly release. Repeat with other leg.
	Standing facing a wall, with hands shoulder height against wall	Walk backwards keeping the heels on the ground until you feel a pull in the calves. Hold for 10.
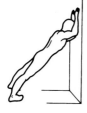	Standing, hands against wall as above	Walk backwards keeping the heels on the ground. When the pull is just being felt, bend the elbows slowly and the pull will increase. Hold for 10.
	Standing on an incline	Lean forward keeping heels on the ground until pull is felt in the calf.
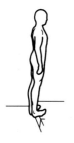	Toe standing on the edge of a step	Lift up onto toes and align body over feet, now lower the heels until the pull is felt in the calf. Hold for 10 then release.
	Reach standing, hands against wall (for soleus only)	Keep the heels on the ground, bend both knees, now take body forward over feet until the pull is felt in the calf. Hold for 10, then release.

Front of thigh stretching: Quadriceps group. Rectus femoris, vastus medialis, vastus lateralis and vastus intermedius

STARTING POSITION	EXERCISE
Support standing	Stand on one leg, grasp the other leg from behind around the ankle. Pull the leg backwards until the pull is felt in front of thigh. Hold for 10 then release. Keep the trunk straight and avoid rotating hip and knee outwards.
Prone lying	Bend right knee towards buttock, grasp ankle and pull until the pull is felt in front of thigh. Hold for 10 then release. Keep the front of the hip joint against the floor.

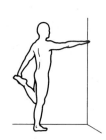

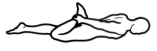

For the fit individual with no back problems, the above exercise can be repeated with both knees bent and pulling on both ankles together.

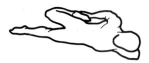

Side lying	Bend one leg, pull heel towards buttocks.
Kneeling	Lean backwards keeping the hips pushed forward until pull is felt in front of thigh. Hold for 10 then sit forward. (*Caution:* not for older clients or for anyone with knee problems.)
Kneeling	Lean backwards, support on hands behind body, push hips forward. Hold for 10 and release. (*Caution:* not for older clients or for anyone with knee problems.)

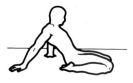

Fit individuals may repeat this exercise using elbow support behind.

Back of thigh stretch: Hamstrings. Biceps femoris, semimembranosus, semitendinosus

STARTING POSITION	EXERCISE
Supine lying with knees at right angle and feet on a wall	Slide right leg up the wall, dorsi flex the foot and tighten the knee. Keeping the leg straight and bottom on the floor, lift the leg away from the wall. Hold for 10 and place back on wall.
Crook lying	Lift right leg up and clasp hands behind the knee. Straighten the knee and dorsi flex the foot until the pull is felt in the back of thigh. Hold for 10 and lower back to crook. (*Caution:* stop if the back arches)
Standing in front of stool or stairs	Place one leg onto the stool or second step of the stairs, reach forward towards the foot keeping the back straight and head in line. Move forward until pull is felt in the back of the thigh. Hold for 10 and release.
Sitting with one leg extended on a plinth.	Straighten back, and lower the trunk onto the thigh.

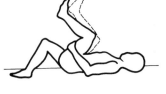

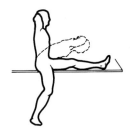

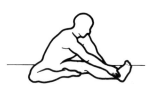

To do the hurdle stretch correctly: Sit on the floor with one leg out in front, bend the other leg and place the foot against inner thigh, role knees out slightly. Then with a straight back and the head in line, lean over the straight leg until a pull is felt in the back of the thigh.

Inner thigh stretching: Adductor group. Adductor longus, adductor magnus, adductor brevis, pectineus and gracilis

STARTING POSITION	EXERCISE
Long sitting	Open legs as far as possible. Keep the back straight and lean forward until pull is felt in the inner thigh. Hold to 10 and release. (*Caution:* do not round the trunk or slouch)
Crook sitting	Keep the feet together and drop knees open as far as possible. Pull the feet towards the body until pull is felt in the inner thigh. Hold for 10 and release. (*Caution:* not to be done by anyone with knee or hip problems)
Crook lying – hands on knees	Part the knees as far as possible, then press apart with hands until pull is felt on the inside of thigh. Hold for 10 and release. (*Caution:* not to be done by anyone with knee or hip problems)
Supine lying with legs up against a wall	Part the legs by sliding along the wall until stretch is felt in the inner thigh. Hold for 10 and release.
Stride standing	Stretch right leg out sideways as far as possible, do not rotate leg outwards. Bend left leg until pull is felt on inner thigh or right leg. Hold for 10 and release.

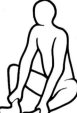
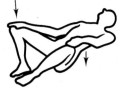
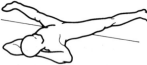

Outer thigh stretch. Hip abductor stretch: Gluteus medius, gluteus minimus, tensor fascia lata

	STARTING POSITION	EXERCISE
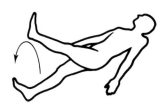	Supine lying	Raise right leg and swing it over the left leg. Lift the right leg slightly and dorsi flex the foot until a pull is felt at outer thigh. Hold for 10 then release.
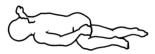	Supine lying	Bend left knee to chest, push the knee across to the right until a pull is felt in the outer thigh, hold for 10 and release.
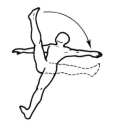	Supine lying	Raise leg to right angle, move across body until pull is felt on the outer thigh.
	Standing	Take the right leg behind the left as far as possible and place foot on the ground with toes turned in. Take the body weight through this leg until a pull is felt in the outer thigh. Hold for 10 then release.
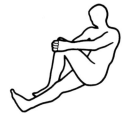	Long sitting	Bend the right knee and place the foot across the left leg level with the knee. Push the bent knee over to the left until a pull is felt in the outer thigh. Hold for 10 and release.

Buttock stretch. Hip extensors: Gluteus maximus

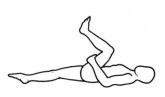

STARTING POSITION	EXERCISE
Lying	Bend right knee onto chest, pull knee closer keeping other leg straight and back flat against floor until a pull is felt in the buttock. Hold for 10 and release.
Inclined prone kneeling	Stretch hands forward onto floor, bend right knee towards hands then drop the trunk onto thigh. Hold for 10 and release. (*Caution:* not to be done by anyone with knee problems)
Standing	Bend right knee to chest, pull knee closer, do not arch the back. Hold for 10 and release. Repeat with other leg.
Standing	Place the right foot on a step, drop the trunk forward and inside the leg, bend left knee until a pull is felt in the right buttock. Hold for 10 and release.
Crook lying	Bend the right lower leg across the left thigh, lift the left leg up and back to apply pressure on the right leg until a pull is felt in the right buttock. Hold for 10 and release.

Hip flexors: Psoas and iliacus, sartorius

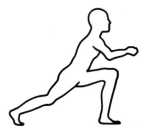

STARTING POSITION	EXERCISE
Walk standing	Bend the forward knee, feeling the pull in the other hip.
Supine lying	Press one leg firmly against the floor and bend other leg onto chest, pull with hands, feel the pull in front of the hip on the straight leg. Hold and release.

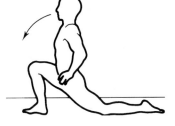

STARTING POSITION	EXERCISE
Half kneeling	Lean forward over the bent knee and feel the pull in the other hip. Hold and release.
On all fours	Lift one leg up behind and place on a chair with knee supported. Bend other knee and let body move downwards, feel the stretch on the straight leg. Hold and release. (*Caution:* not to be done by anyone with a knee problem)
Crook lying	Lift buttocks off the floor, push upwards as high as possible. Hold and release.

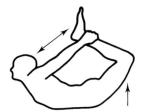

STARTING POSITION	EXERCISE
Prone lying	Bend knees and grasp feet with hands, pull trunk up. Hold and release. (*Caution:* should only be done by the young and flexible)

Lower back stretch: Erector spinae and quadratus lumborum

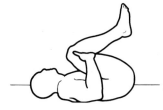

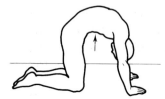

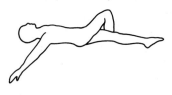

STARTING POSITION	EXERCISE
Crook lying	Press small of back into the floor, bring right knee onto chest, clasp hands around the knee and pull towards chest. Hold then relax.
Crook lying	Press small of back into floor, bring both knees onto chest, clasp hands around thighs and pull towards chest. Hold for 10 and release.
Crook lying	As above but also lift head and shoulders off the ground. Hold for 10 and release.
Crook lying	Keep the knees together and drop down to the right, feeling the pull on left side. Hold and release. Then drop the knees to the other side. Hold and release.
Yard lying	Bend right knee and place foot outside the left knee. Bring the left hand down and pull the knee to the left, keep the right arm and shoulder on floor. Hold and release.
Prone kneeling	Contract the abdominals and round the back, lower to the horizontal.
Crook lying – place a firm rolled towel under the sacrum	Press the lower back against the floor. Hold and release.
Sitting, feet on floor	Lean the body forward, taking the trunk down to thigh. Hang the arms to side.

Arm stretching: biceps, triceps

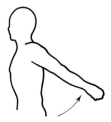

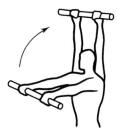

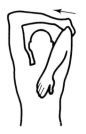

STARTING POSITION	EXERCISE
Biceps – stride standing	Clasp the hands behind the back, keep the elbows straight, raise arms upwards. Hold for 10 and release.
Biceps – stride standing	Lift a bar above the head and stretch backwards. Keep elbows straight.
Triceps – stride standing	Lift the right arm upwards and bend the elbow so that the hand lies behind the head. Use the other hand behind the head to push the upper arm down further.
Triceps – stride standing	Clasp the hands above the head, and pull the arms over as far as possible behind the head. Hold for 10 and release.
Latissimus dorsi stretch – stride standing	Lift the arm upwards and bend the elbow so that the hand lies behind the head. Use the other hand to pull the arm towards body and bend the trunk to the same side. Hold and release.
Stretch stride standing	Place back of hands together, stretch towards ceiling.

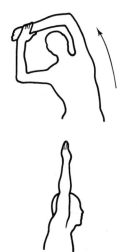

Front of thorax: Pectoralis major stretch

STARTING POSITION	EXERCISE
Stride standing	Press the shoulders backwards.
Crook lying arms at sides	Place a tightly rolled hand towel lengthways between the scapulae. Press the shoulders down into the floor.
Crook lying arms out to side, elbows at right angles, palms facing upwards	The same action as above.
Yard crook lying	The same action as above.
Prone kneeling	Stretch the arms forward and outwards until the elbows are straight. Extend the wrist and drop the chest forward, pulling the shoulders backwards.
Lying with a pillow between the shoulders	Raise the arms above the head and press them into the floor.
Stride standing or High sitting	Place one bent arm upwards behind head, and the other bent arm downward behind back. Clasp the hands if possible or link them with a towel or strap. Pull downwards, bringing the upper arm back and nearer the head. Repeat with other arm.
Stride standing or High sitting	Use a bar which is shoulder width long or just over. Hold the bar at the end, lift upwards above head and then downwards behind head.

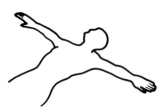

Long sitting in front of chair or wall bars	Place arms behind and grasp the sides of the chair. Keep the elbows straight and thrust the chest upwards and forwards, keeping the chin in. Hold then release.
Standing with back to wall bars	Place arms behind and grasp the wall bar just below shoulder height. Drop the body forward and pull back between scapulae. Keep the chin in. Hold and release.
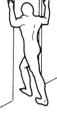 Walk standing in an open doorway	With the elbows and shoulders at right angles, place one hand on the wall on either side of the doorway. Lean forward into the doorway.

Questions

1 Explain what is meant by 'the flexibility' of a joint.
2 Give three reasons why flexibility is important to an athlete.
3 Briefly explain the six factors which influence flexibility.
4 Give the two ranges of movement through which a joint must be exercised to maintain and improve flexibility.
5 Explain three reasons why ballistic stretching is not recommended.
6 Explain the following terms:
  A active stretching
  B active assisted stretching
  C passive stretching
7 List six effects of stretch training.
8 State where 'the pull' should be felt during static stretching.
9 Explain when the stretching phase should be performed within a training programme.

CHAPTER 10

Rest and Relaxation

Rest and relaxation are important considerations for all those involved in fitness training. Rest allows the tissues to recover and the body systems to return to a balanced state. It is important that homeostasis is restored, otherwise the body will become progressively over stressed and will fail to function efficiently.

Rest

Strength training involves overloading the muscles to near breakdown. They then repair, adapt and grow during the rest period. If this rest period is inadequate, adaptation and growth will not take place and there will be little or no strength gains. At least 48 hours of rest should be allowed between sessions. Maximum lifters may allow five to seven days' rest; they may train every day, using different muscles.

Endurance athletes rest to ensure that stores of glycogen are built up within the muscles and liver. Rest is essential following injury to allow for full recovery of the tissues. The duration of rest will depend on the extent of the injury. Rest does not necessarily mean a complete cessation of activity; it may mean that the overload is considerably reduced. Exercising at a much lower level of intensity will allow gradual recovery from intense activity. Training can be planned to stress alternative systems, and allow the recovery of others.

Relaxation

The ability to relax combats stress, tension and anxiety. Stress affects body balance (homeostasis), and the body fails to function efficiently, resulting in fatigue, lethargy, illness and disease. Stressors (factors causing stress) may be extrinsic or intrinsic. They may be social, chemical, bacterial, physical, climactic, or psychological. People differ in their ability to cope with stress; some are more affected than others.

The symptoms of stress are easily identifiable eg, increased sweating, increased heart rate, increased blood pressure, rapid breathing, dryness of the mouth, inability to cope, feeling overwhelmed and out of control, inability to concentrate or make decisions, trembling, nail biting, frequent urination, non-stop talking, pacing and other nervous habits.

It is impossible to remove all stressors from daily life; in fact, a certain degree of stress is desirable, productive, and can produce feelings of thrill and excitement.

Many athletes suffer psychological stresses prior to competition. This competitive anxiety may manifest itself as:

1 cognitive anxiety or mental worry: eg, 'I'm not ready', 'I have not trained well enough' and other negative thoughts.
2 somatic anxiety or physiological symptoms such as 'I feel sick', 'my muscles are tense'.

Stress and anxiety may adversely affect performance but it can be directed towards enhancing it. The athlete must focus on his goal and learn to cope and control negative feelings. Some are better at this than others, which gives them the edge during performance.

The ability to relax at the right moment is crucial for the athlete. Regular practice of relaxation techniques will reduce anxiety, conserve energy, reduce fatigue, lethargy and overtiredness, and aid recovery.

Aids to relaxation

A variety of aids can be used to promote relaxation. These are not however always to hand, and are not essential.

- Heat therapy, eg, heat packs, heat blankets, hot baths, showers, sauna and steam baths and infra red lamps.
- Cold therapy, eg, cold packs and wraps.
- Massage performed in a deep slow and rhythmical manner.

■ Analgesic liniments, wintergreen and other muscle relaxants (drugs are also used in certain circumstances).

Preparation of room for relaxation

The selection of a warm, quiet environment and the positioning and comfort of the client are important considerations. These factors alone may be sufficient to illicit the relaxation response (see page 179).

■ The area should be warm and well ventilated.
■ The area should be quiet and away from any distracting noises or activities.
■ The lighting should be low and well diffused.
■ The colour scheme should be soft and warming, using pastel rather than bold colours.
■ The area should be spotlessly clean and tidy. All linen and towels should be boil-washed and well laundered.
■ A comfortable mattress on the floor provides the best support, with pillows for the head and knees. Two low plinths pushed together and covered with a thin mattress can be used. (Clients feel more secure nearer the ground and on a wide rather than narrow surface.) Reclining chairs are also suitable.
■ Light blankets can be used for additional warmth.
■ Very soft relaxing music may be played in the background as some clients do not like absolute quiet and will become tense. This will depend on client preference.

Client care

A full client consultation should be carried out.

■ Allow the client time to discuss their lifestyle and any problems which may be contributing to stress and anxiety levels.
■ Discuss stress levels at work or during sport or training, which may be affecting performance. Advise and suggest strategies for coping where possible. Explain how relaxation will help.
■ Suggest suitable clothing such as loose fitting cotton vest, T shirt, sweater and loose fitting pyjama or track suit bottoms; loose socks can be worn on the feet. (Do not

allow the client to walk around in socks, as there is a danger of slipping.)

■ If suitable clothing is not available, loosen clothing, remove tie and belt, loosen collar and trousers or skirt and remove shoes.

■ Suggest that the client uses the toilet beforehand as it is impossible to relax with a full bladder.

■ Use some form of heat if available prior to the commencement of relaxation training. (Follow the correct procedure when applying heat – see page 295.)

■ Create an atmosphere conducive to relaxation. Smile, be calm, pleasant and relaxed, speak slowly and clearly, keep your voice low, do not rush or hurry the client. Explain the procedure clearly and carefully to alleviate any anxiety.

Examples of relaxation techniques

To achieve long-term benefits, the individual must be taught to recognise the difference between being in a tense state and being in a relaxed state. As physical and mental relaxation are interdependent, both areas must be trained. Although relaxation techniques may appear simple, they are skills which must be learnt and practised regularly.

■ The relaxation response.
■ Progressive relaxation (contract, relax technique).
■ Visualisation or imagery.
■ Biofeedback.

The relaxation response

This is the client's response to four basic conditions: a quiet environment, a comfortable position, a mental image to concentrate on, and a passive attitude.

1 *A quiet environment* – this cuts out noise and limits distraction; it allows the individual to switch off.

2 *A comfortable position* – the position selected for all relaxation techniques is very important. The body must be totally supported so that muscle tension is reduced. The position should be selected to suit the preference of the client; lying, half lying or recovery position may be chosen. The body must be well supported with pillows to minimise muscle effort and enable the client to remain in this position for a considerable length of time.

3 *Mental concentration* – this can be an image to concentrate on such as a sphere, box, vase etc., or it may be any object in the room such as a clock or plain curtain. The client concentrates hard on this one image and empties the mind of other thoughts or images.

4 *A passive attitude* – this is the most difficult, especially for those with extreme mental anxiety. It involves letting go and emptying the mind of thoughts and distractions.

Progressive relaxation

This method was developed by Dr Edmund Jacobson, one of the pioneers in the field of relaxation. It aims to develop an awareness of the difference between feelings of tension and those of relaxation, within muscles and muscle groups. The client is taught to contract and relax each muscle group in sequence from the foot to the head. With practice, the client will appreciate the difference between being tense and being relaxed, and will develop the ability to quickly adopt the relaxed state. Following this, the client can be taught to recognise differing degrees of tension within muscles by using the same sequence but varying the contraction; from full contraction, then part contraction, to minimal contraction for each muscle or group.

TECHNIQUE

- Select a suitable venue and prepare the client.
- The client should lie on the mattress or be fully supported in a reclining chair. Any modification of lying can be used; eg, the recovery position with the body well supported with pillows; the supine position (on the back) with a pillow under the head and knees; half lying with a pillow for the head and knees. Encourage the client to 'let go', breathe deeply and close the eyes gently, before carrying out the following instructions.
- Begin with the feet and repeat each movement three times.
  Pull feet up (dorsi flexion) hard then let go.
  Push feet down (plantar flexion) hard then let go.
  Push knees down hard against floor then let go.
  Push leg down hard against floor then let go.
  Tighten buttock muscles hard then let go.
  Pull tummy in hard and then let go.
  Raise shoulders off floor then let go.
  Press shoulders into floor hard then let go.
  Press arms into floor hard then let go.

Curl fingers to make a fist then let go.
Press head into floor then let go.
Screw up and tighten the face then let go.
Tighten all groups then let go.

- The therapist must use the voice to good effect when teaching relaxation. The command 'tighten hard' should be firm and held out and then 'let go' should be a lower tone and held out longer to encourage the feeling of letting go. The terms 'relax', 'release' can be used or interchanged with 'let go'.
- The client should breathe out as she 'lets go'.
- Clients can then practise the sequence on their own until they are free of tension and sleepy. They should be left for 15–20 minutes and then woken up slowly.

As clients develop the ability to relax, they can be taught to appreciate differing degrees of tension. This is done in the same way as above except that the first contraction must be maximal, the second contraction partial and the third contraction minimal. The commands would be as follows:

1 Pull the feet up hard, hard, hard and relax.
2 Gently pull the feet up, just feel the muscle pulling and relax.
3 Just move the foot upwards ever so slightly and relax.
4 Practise the three different contractions again in your own time – feel the difference in muscle tension each time.

Work through the body in this way, using the same sequence as above.

Visualisation or imagery

This technique requires the individual to visualise situations or conditions conducive to relaxation; eg:

- Imagine lying on the beach in warm sunshine. It is quiet and peaceful, you feel warm and heavy.
- Imagine lying in a field in warm sunshine, you smell the grass, feel warm and heavy.
- Imagine sinking into a feather duvet, it feels soft and warm and wraps around you.
- Think of any situation which recalls warmth, comfort and peace.
- Concentrate entirely on the rhythm of breathing, let breathing become deeper and slower.

Any examples that enhance relaxation can be included.

VISUALISATION WITH RELAXATION AND BREATHING

This can be practised on your own, in any comfortable well supported position.

- Imagine any pleasing situation such as those above.
- Breathe deeply and slowly.
- Concentrate on different parts of the body in turn and feel the tension flow away; eg, think of your head and face, let the tension flow away, your head feels heavy, your jaw feels heavy, let go, breathe deeply and slowly.
- Repeat this process for each area of the body.

Visualisation and breathing can be used to good effect when performing stretch/flexibility exercises which require the relaxed state.

Biofeedback

When it is difficult to appreciate the difference between muscle tension and relaxation, techniques of biofeedback may be used using special equipment. These devices give a reading which relates to the degree of tension and the mind is then used to attempt a change in the reading.

Questions

1 List some aids which may be used to promote relaxation.
2 Explain why rest is important between training sessions.
3 Explain the factors which must be considered when preparing the room for relaxation.
4 List four basic conditions which promote the relaxation response.
5 Describe the positioning of the client prior to teaching relaxation.
6 Describe briefly how you would teach progressive relaxation technique.
7 Explain how breathing and visualisation may be used to promote relaxation.
8 Briefly explain the effect of inadequate rest and relaxation on the sportsperson.

CHAPTER II

Posture

Posture is the term used to describe the alignment of the body, ie, how the body is held. Good posture means that the body is balanced and the muscle work required to maintain it is minimal. Poor posture means that the body is out of balance and certain muscles must contract strongly to maintain it; over time, those muscles will tighten and shorten, while others weaken and stretch. This muscle imbalance imposes stresses on the underlying structures, the ligaments and joints, resulting in deformities, stiffness and pain. Certain muscles are unable to work through their full range, the body loses its ability to function at maximum efficiency, and the performance of activities, movement and exercise (as well as the activities of daily living) can become severely limited.

The effects of good and bad posture

Poor alignment of one part of the body can affect other parts. This can be more clearly understood if we think of the body in terms of segments. Each segment must be perfectly balanced on the other. If one segment moves forward, backwards or sideways, adjustments have to be made in all the other segments for balance to be restored. Good posture is important to the athlete or sportsman as it decreases muscle strain and allows the body to function at maximum efficiency.

Poor posture affects general health. The natural movements of the thorax are restricted, its expansion is limited which results in shallow breathing. This reduces the intake of oxygen and elimination of carbon dioxide. The circulation is affected due to the tension in muscles and reduction in thoracic movement. Blood is unable to flow as freely around the body. This limits delivery of nutrients and elimination of waste products.

Posture is dynamic, constantly adjusting to counteract the forces acting upon the body. Postural adjustments may be made consciously or unconsciously. The cerebral cortex, basal nuclei, cerebellum and brain stem all play a part in the control of posture. These higher centres respond to different impulses passing in from various sensory receptors. Information on the body's position in space is received from muscle spindles, tendon and joint receptors, from the eyes, the ears and from the skin on the soles of the feet. The higher centres respond to incoming information and relay impulses back to muscles, initiating their contraction to take corrective action.

Influences on posture

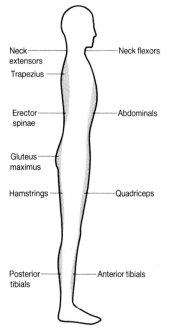

Figure 11.1   *Postural muscles*

Posture is influenced by many factors, both physical and psychological. A large percentage of the population lead sedentary lifestyles and take little exercise, which leads to muscle imbalance and poor body alignment. Other factors which influence posture include:

- hereditary weight distribution
- height
- tension
- illness
- fatigue
- occupational stresses
- poor working conditions
- poor sitting positions.

Psychological and emotional states also have an effect – those who are happy, confident, extrovert with high self esteem, exhibit good posture, while those who are unhappy, sad, introverted, lacking in confidence and with low self esteem generally have poor posture.

The importance of good posture

Good postural habits should be developed when young and maintained throughout life. It is possible to improve posture for all age groups through appropriate exercise. The extent of the improvement will depend on the degree of deformity, the age and the commitment of the individual. Good posture is important for the following reasons:

- Maintaining muscle balance.
- Improving body shape and appearance.
- Preventing muscle tension, spasm and pain.

- Preventing stresses on ligaments, tendons and joints.
- Preventing skeletal deformities and associated pain.
- Increasing movement of the thorax, resulting in deeper breathing with increase in oxygen intake and elimination of carbon dioxide.
- Improving the efficiency of the circulatory system.
- Improving the performance of all activities and exercises and enhancing peak performance.
- Reducing the risk of musculo-skeletal injuries.

Evaluation of posture

Posture must be accurately examined and evaluated before correction can take place; this should form part of any pre-exercise consultation. All findings should be carefully recorded and appropriate exercises devised for correction of the faults.

Aids to postural assessment

The following aids can be used to make assessment easier and accurate.

- A plumb line to check body alignment.
- A mirror to provide visual feedback for the client. First, look at 'normal' posture and discuss problem areas with the client. Correct the posture and discuss the improvements. View from the front, side and back. On the front view, lines can be drawn to check the level of ear lobes, shoulders, waist angles, anterior, superior, iliac spines and knees.
- A graphed board can be used: the client stands in front of the board and the relevant bony points marked – ear lobes, shoulders, waist angles, knees – and examined for any deviation and discussed.

It is not necessary to use all these aids but one or two will help the client to appreciate his/her problems.

Examination of posture

If possible, observe posture as the client walks around the room (this may not be possible in a small cubicle). Many problems can be observed when the body is in motion. Observe the posture when sitting down and standing up; are movements evenly balanced or does the client sit and stand unevenly?

Ask the client to adopt his/her normal stance and assess the posture from the front, side and back.

From the front

HEAD POSITION

- Are the ear lobes level? If not, there is muscle imbalance. The sterno-cleido mastoid and upper fibres of trapezius are tight on the lower side; those on the other side will be stretched.

SHOULDERS

- Are they level, or is one higher than the other? This would indicate muscle imbalance. The upper fibres of trapezius and levator scapulae are tight on the raised side. A difference in level may also indicate scoliosis (a slight difference is considered normal).
- Are both shoulders held high? This indicates tension in the muscles on both sides. The right and left upper fibres of trapezius and levator scapulae are tight.
- Are the shoulders drawn forwards, and rounded? This indicates muscle imbalance. The pectoral muscles are tight but the middle fibres of trapezius and the rhomboids are stretched.
- Are there hollows above the clavicles? This indicates muscle tension which may be due to respiratory problems such as asthma.

BREASTS

- Are breasts held high or sagging? If there is breast sag and round shoulders, correction of posture may help to lift the breasts.

WAIST

- Are the waist angles on the right side and left side level? If one is lower than the other, there may be spinal deformity or a difference in leg length.

ANTERIOR SUPERIOR ILIAC SPINES

- Are they level? If not, there may be spinal deformity or a difference in leg length.
- Are they dropped forward? This indicates a lordosis with

tight erector spinae, quadratus lumborum and weak
abdominals.

■ Are they dropped backwards? This indicates flat back or
sway back with weak back extensors; ie, erector spinae
and quadratus lumborum and tight abdominals.

THE PATELLAE

■ Do they point forward? If not, there may be knock knees
(genu valgum) or bow legs (genu varum).

THE TOES

■ Do they point forward? If not, do they point outward?
There may be flattening of the medial arch and flat feet.

■ If they point inwards or outwards, the weight distribution
over the foot will be wrong and will cause foot problems.

■ Look for bunions where the big toe deviates towards and
sometimes across the other toes, and there is swelling at
the metatarsophalangeal joint.

■ Look for hammer toes where the interphalangeal joints
are deformed.

From the side

Use a plumb line – this should fall through the lobe of the
ear, the point of the shoulder through the hip joint, behind
the patella and just in front of the lateral malleolus.

HEAD POSITION

■ Is the neck or cervical curve exaggerated and the chin
forward? This means that the neck extensors and upper
fibres of trapezius at the back of the neck are tight, and
the neck flexors are weak.

THORACIC CURVE

■ Is there kyphosis, ie, an exaggerated thoracic curve,
giving a humped look? This means that the pectoral
muscles are tight and the middle fibres of trapezius and
rhomboids are weak.

ABDOMEN

■ Is the abdomen protruding or sagging forwards,
indicating weakness of the abdominal muscles? The
pelvis will tilt forward.

LUMBAR CURVE

■ Is there lordosis (ie, an exaggerated lumbar curve with
the spine curved inwards)? This means that there will be

an anterior pelvis tilt with weak abdominals and tight erector spinae, quadratus lumborum, hip flexors (psoas and iliacus).

■ If the lumbar region is flat which is much less common, the erector spinae and quadratus lumborum will be weak.

BUTTOCKS

■ Are the buttocks well toned with strong muscles, or are the gluteal muscles weak and sagging?

KNEES

■ Are the knees hyper extended?

From the back

HEAD

■ Are the ear lobes level, or is the head tilted indicating muscle imbalance?

SHOULDERS

■ Are they level (see page 186)?
■ Is there winged scapula (ie, the inferior angle and medial border of the scapula lifting away from the chest wall)? This indicates a weakness of serratus anterior and lower fibres of trapezius.

SPINE

■ Is there scoliosis (ie, a lateral deviation of the spine? This may be an S or C curve to the right or left. (If you are unsure, pull a finger firmly down the spinous processes; the red line will show up any deviation, as the line should be straight.) A scoliosis may be structural (being born that way), or it may be postural, which will straighten out when the body is flexed forward.

BUTTOCKS

■ Are the buttock folds level? If they are not, scoliosis, lateral pelvic tilt or different leg length may be present.

HEELS

■ Are these square and firmly planted on the ground? If not, the weight distribution will be uneven.

Correction of posture

Feet

The correction of posture should begin at the feet. Stand with the feet 4–6 inches apart, toes pointing forward. The weight should be evenly distributed between the balls of the feet and the heels.

Practise the following:

- Raise the toes off ground, feel weight evenly between balls and heels, then lower toes.
- Sway body forward, feel more weight on balls of the feet.
- Sway body backward, feel more weight on heels.
- Position body so that the weight is evenly distributed between balls and heels.
- Lift the medial arch slightly but do not curl the toes.

Knees

- Press knees backwards (hard) and then ease the knees by bending slightly; find mid point and pull knee caps upwards.
- If the knees are hyper extended, ease them slightly and pull knee caps upwards as above.
- If the knees are bowed or knock kneed, tighten the kneecaps, rotate the thighs outwards and tighten the buttocks to bring the knee caps to point forward.

(Check feet again.)

Pelvis

Tilt the pelvis forward and then backwards, pull the abdomen in again, tucking the tail under and hold this balance. (Pull the abdomen in and breathe out as the pelvis is pulled forward, then hold this position while breathing normally.)

Thorax

Pull the thorax upwards from the waist as you breathe in, drawing the shoulders backwards and downwards. (Hold while breathing normally. Do not thrust the chest forwards.)

Neck and head

■ Elongate the neck, pull the chin backwards. Feel as though someone is pulling the hair upwards at the crown.

Check feet, knees, pelvis and thorax again, hold this position then relax.

Practise this correction several times a day and during various activities; correct posture during inhalation, and hold balance during exhalation. A stiff military posture is not desirable – relax a little. Walk around holding the new posture, and it will eventually become habitual.

Corrective exercises for postural problems

After the problem has been diagnosed, the objectives of treatment must be clearly stated and explained to the client. The client must be encouraged to practise the exercises at home.

Below are suggested exercises for the correction of common problems. Read the sections on strengthening and stretching, warm up and cool down. Any appropriate exercises may be selected from those listed, or you may add some of your own. Remember that strength will only improve if the muscle is made to work progressively harder.

Postural correction of lordosis

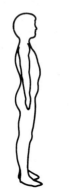

This is an exaggerated curve of the lumbar spine and the pelvis is tilted forward. The weak muscles that require strengthening are

■ the abdominals: rectus abdominus, internal oblique and the external oblique
■ the hip extensors: the hamstrings and gluteus maximus.

The tight muscles which require stretching are

■ the trunk extensors: erector spinae and quadratus lumborum
■ the hip flexors, particularly ilio psoas.

Figure 11.2   *Lordosis*

Aims of treatment

- to strengthen the abdominals, thus pulling the pelvis upwards
- to strengthen the hip extensors
- to stretch erector spinae and quadratus lumborum
- to stretch the hip flexors.

Remember to use crook lying as a starting position for the abdominal strengthening, and to keep the small of the back against the floor.

Lordosis – sample scheme

Warm up

Choose exercises from schemes on page 213.

Main corrective exercises

Crook lying	Pelvic roll, press lumbar region into floor, release.
Crook lying	Chin in, raise head and shoulders to look at knees.
Crook lying	Curl up.

(This will be progressed by moving hand position to head rest, and then stretch above head.)

Bend crook lying	Twist, bringing alternate elbow to opposite knee.
Yard crook lying	Drop knees to right then left.
Lying	Slide right arm down right side and left arm down left side.
Prone kneeling	Arch back to stretch the lumbar spine, returning to horizontal.
Prone kneeling	Stretch alternate legs out and up 15% from horizontal.

Cool down

Yard lying	Bend right knee and place foot outside left knee. Bring left hand down and pull bent knee to the left.

	Keep right arm and shoulder on the floor. Hold for 10 then release. Repeat other side.
Crook lying	Place a firm rolled towel under the sacrum. Press the lower back against the floor. Hold for 10 then release.
Half kneeling	Lean forward over bent knee and feel a pull in the front of the opposite hip. Hold for 10 and release.
Stride standing	Pull in abdomen and release.
Stride standing	Pelvic rotations.
Gentle jogging	Arm swinging.
Lying	Deep breathing: pull in abdomen as you exhale.

Postural correction of kyphosis

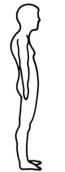

This is an exaggerated curve of the thoracic region: the shoulders are usually rounded, the neck is shortened and held in extension and the chin pokes forward.

■ The weak muscles that require strengthening are the middle fibres of trapezius, the rhomboids and erector spinae.
■ The tight muscles that require stretching are pectoralis major and the neck extensors.

Figure 11.3   *Kyphosis*

Aims of treatment

■ to strengthen the shoulder retractors (namely middle fibres of trapezius and the rhomboids), thus drawing the shoulders backwards
■ to strengthen erector spinae to maintain the erect posture
■ to stretch pectoralis major.

Remember that many of these exercises are also used to correct round shoulders. Always keep the chin in and maintain a long neck when performing these exercises.

Kyphosis – sample scheme

Warm up
Choose exercises from schemes on page 213.

Main corrective exercises

Standing	Posture correction – hold.
Stride standing	Gently drop the head forward. Pull chin in, press head back making a long neck. Raise.
Lax stoop sitting	Raise trunk gradually from below, vertebra by vertebra.
Lax stoop sitting	As above, against resistance from therapist.
Stride standing	Circle shoulders backwards.
Stride standing	Circle arms backwards.
Stride standing	Pull shoulders backwards.
Across bend stride standing	Pull shoulders back, release. Pull elbows back, release. Press arms back, release.
Lax stoop stride standing	Slowly return to standing, from below, vertebra by vertebra.
Stoop standing	Clasp hands behind back. Pull arms and shoulders up and back. Hold for 10 and release.
Prone lying (face down)	Chin in, pull shoulders back. Raise head and shoulders.
Prone lying, hands clasped behind back	Pull on hands and pull shoulders off the floor.
Prone lying, hands clasped behind back	Chin in, pull shoulders back, lift head and shoulders.
Wing prone lying	Chin in, lift head and shoulders off the floor. Pull shoulders back.

Wing prone lying	As above, against resistance of the therapist.
Prone lying	Arms abducted, elbows bent, palms to floor. Lift arms and head and shoulders.
Yard prone lying	As above.

Cool down

Crook lying	Place a tightly rolled towel lengthways along the spine between the scapulae. Press the shoulders back towards the floor. Hold for 10 and release.
Crook lying, arms out to side, elbows at right angles, palms facing forward	Same action as above.
Yard crook lying	Same action as above.
Sitting	Place one arm upwards behind the head and the other down behind the back. Clasp hands or link with a strap pull downwards, bringing the upper arm nearer the head. Hold for 10 and release.
Sitting	Use a bar at least shoulder width long. Hold the bar with hands, shoulder width apart. Lift bar upwards above the head and then down behind the head. Hold for 10 and lift up.
Prone kneeling	Raise alternate arms side ways and upwards.
Gentle jog	Arm circling backwards.
Walk around	Arm swinging.

Kypho-lordosis is a combination of the previous two conditions. Select exercises from the two schemes for this condition.

Postural correction of round shoulders

The shoulders are protracted (drawn forward), the head is extended and the chin pokes forward. This postural defect may be present without any problem with the spine (ie, kyphosis). However, if the spine is kyphotic, the shoulders will also be rounded.

- The weak muscles which require strengthening are the middle fibres of trapezius and the rhomboids.
- The tight muscles which require stretching are the pectorals and neck extensors.

Aims of treatment

- to strengthen the shoulder retractors and draw the shoulders backwards
- to stretch pectoralis major and neck extensors.

For suitable exercises, refer to the scheme for kyphosis. The same exercises can be used for both conditions. You may wish to modify this slightly by adding your own.

Postural correction of scoliosis

This is a lateral curvature of the spine. It may be a long C curve or an S curve. This condition may cause scapular deviation, slight uneven levels of the shoulder and pelvic girdle, caused by muscle imbalance on the right and left side of the spine.

The spine must be carefully examined. To make observation easier, pull a finger downwards with slight pressure along the spinous processes. The red line will show the extent and direction of the curve. If the condition is postural, the curve will right itself in forward flexion. Ask the client to bend over; if the condition does not correct with flexion, it is a structural problem and should be referred to a doctor.

- The muscles that require strengthening will be the ones on the outside of the curve.
- The muscles that require stretching will be on the inside of the curve.

General back strengthening exercises are usually effective in correcting this condition. It is frequently found in adolescence when pupils carry heavy school bags over the same shoulder or in the same hand each day. Suggest that the bag is carried in one hand to school or work, and the other on the way home.

Aims of the treatment

- to restore balance to muscles of the back, thus reducing the deformity.

Scoliosis – sample scheme

Warm up

Choose exercises from schemes on page 213.

Corrective exercises

Stride standing	Reach up into the air, with the hand on the concave side of the curve where the muscles are tight. Reach towards the floor with the other hand. Stretch, hold, relax, repeat.
Stride standing	Trunk side flexion to the convex side where the muscles are stretched. Slide the hand down the side and return.
Prone lying	As above, but reach arm up along the floor on concave side and slide arm down the side of convexity. Hold, release and repeat.
Prone lying	Stretch arm above head and opposite leg along floor.
Prone lying	Raise opposite arm and leg as above.
Crook lying	Arms abducted and elbows at right angles, palms to floor. Rotate arms to palms up and push back into floor.
Prone lying	Arms abducted and elbows at right angles palms to floor. Raise arms backwards.

Prone lying, arms to side	Chin in, lift head and shoulders.
Prone lying, clasp hands	Chin in, lift head and shoulders and pull down the arms.
Prone lying	Arms abducted, elbows at right angles, palms to floor. Raise arms head and shoulders (do not extend the head; keep in line with the body).
Yard prone lying	As above.
Stretch prone lying	As above.

Cool down

Select from previous schemes; include plenty of shoulder and trunk movements.

Postural correction of flat back

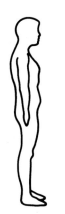

This is a condition where there is little or no lumbar curve, the back is flat in this region and the pelvis is tilted backwards. It is usually accompanied by kyphosis of the thoracic spine.

■ The muscles that require strengthening are the back extensors, ie, erector spinae (sometimes the abdominals are weak and so is gluteus maximus).
■ The muscles that require stretching are the hamstrings.

Figure 11.4   *Flat back*

Aims of the treatment

■ to try and develop a normal lumbar curve by strengthening erector spinae and gluteus maximus
■ to maintain correct pelvic tilt by ensuring strength of the abdominals and stretch of the hamstrings.

Flat back – sample scheme

Warm up
Choose exercises from schemes on page 213.

Corrective exercises

Sitting	Lean forward, taking pressure from buttocks onto thigh. Now extend back to create a lumbar lordosis. Hold for 10 and return.
Prone lying	Alternate leg raise.
Prone lying	Double leg raise.
Prone kneeling	Arch back and hollow.
Prone kneeling	Lift alternate leg up and backwards. Stretch and hold, return.
Lying with rolled towel under lumbar spine	Flex one knee then extend the leg up towards the ceiling. Keep the opposite leg hard down on the floor. Repeat other leg.
Long sitting	Rotate pelvis forward then lean slightly backwards. Hold and return.
Supine lying with legs up against a wall, towel under lumbar spine	Pull alternate legs away from the wall, keeping the knee straight, keep the pelvis on the floor. Hold and return.

Cool down
Select from previous schemes

Correction of winged scapula

This is a condition where the medial border and inferior angle of the scapula move back away from the chest wall. It is due to weakness of serratus anterior and lower fibres of trapezius.

- Muscles that require strengthening are serratus anterior and lower fibres of trapezius.

Aims of treatment

- To strengthen those muscles which hold the scapula against the chest wall.

Remember that serratus anterior is used powerfully in all punching movements. It helps trapezius to swing the scapula laterally during arm abduction and swinging, and it works powerfully to hold the scapula in position when the weight of the body is taken on the hands, as in prone kneeling, push ups and press ups.

Winged scapula – sample scheme

Warm up
Choose exercises from schemes on page 213.

Main corrective exercises

Bend, stride standing	Punch forward, punch pillow or punch bag.
Stride standing	Hands against therapist, elbows bent. Push alternate arms straight against therapist's resistance.
Bend stride standing or sitting	Arm stretch vertically upwards. Repeat with progressive weights.
Stride standing, arms bent, wall leaning	Push away from the wall.
Prone kneeling	Bend and straighten elbows.
Prone lying	Hands under shoulders, push ups.
Prone lying	Press ups.
Crook lying	Hold weight in hands at shoulders, push weights vertically upwards and lower. Weights can be increased for progression.

Cool down
Select from previous schemes.

Questions

1 Give six effects of poor posture.
2 Describe the use of any two 'aids' which may be used when assessing posture.
3 List all the points that a plumb line must pass through, if posture is correct.
4 Describe the postural problem 'kyphosis', indicate which muscles are involved.
5 Name the condition associated with anterior pelvic tilt.

6 Give six exercises for the correction of each of the following conditions:
  A round shoulders
  B lordosis
  C flat back.
7 Name the weak muscles associated with 'winged scapula', give four exercises to strengthen these muscles.

CHAPTER 12

Starting Positions and Exercise Routines

The starting position for exercises must be included when writing exercise schemes. Lengthy descriptions of these positions can be avoided by using the abbreviated standard terminology listed below. When compiling schemes, two columns should be used: one for the starting position and the other giving instructions for the exercises.

This chapter also includes examples of mobility exercises, warm up and cool down exercises and a section on how to teach breathing exercises.

Starting positions

When writing out exercise schemes, it is vital to state the starting position as it influences the muscle work and the stability of the body. Younger clients may be safe and stable in standing positions, but older clients are more stable and feel safer in sitting or lying. Older clients or those with arthritis or joint problems should not be placed in the kneeling position.

There are five basic starting positions:

- lying (also known as supine lying)
- kneeling
- sitting
- standing
- hanging.

Modifications of starting positions

Modifications of these basic positions are made to increase or decrease the difficulty of the exercise. Modifications are made to:

- raise or lower the centre of gravity
- increase or decrease the size of the base, thus changing stability
- increase or decrease leverage
- provide adequate fixation of the body so that specific movements can be performed with maximum concentration
- increase or decrease the muscle work required to maintain the position
- ensure maximum support for relaxation.

The five basic starting positions can be modified as below:

1 *Lying:* prone lying, side lying, half lying, crook lying, crook lying with pelvis lifted.

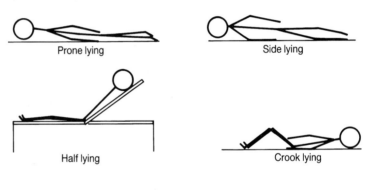

Figure 12.1   *Modifications of lying*

2 *Kneeling:* prone kneeling, inclined prone kneeling, heel sitting, half kneeling.

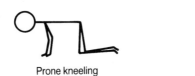

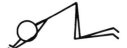

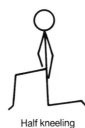

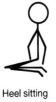

Figure 12.2 *Modifications of kneeling*

3 *Sitting:* crook sitting, long sitting, astride sitting, side sitting, stoop sitting, fall out sitting.

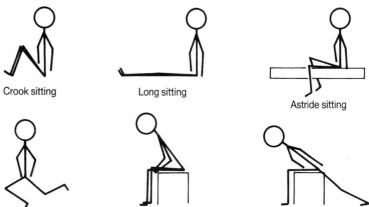

Figure 12.3 *Modifications of sitting*

4 *Standing:* toe standing, stride standing, walk standing, step standing.

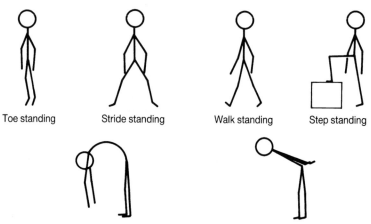

Figure 12.4 *Modifications of standing*

5 *Hanging:* stride hanging, knee bend hanging.

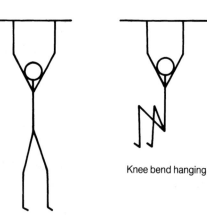

Figure 12.5 *Modifications of hanging*

The position of the arms is also very important and these are usually written first, eg, *bend* stride standing.

- *Arm positions:* wing, low wing, bend, across bend, under bend, reach, yard, stretch, head rest.

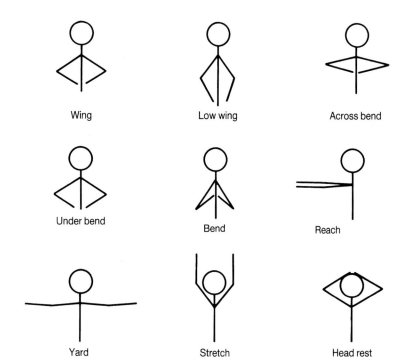

Figure 12.6   *Arm position*

Mobility exercises

These are safe exercises that are practised to maintain mobility in joints. A selection may be included as appropriate in exercise classes.

Neck mobility

(Keep the shoulders relaxed throughout)

STARTING POSITION	EXERCISE
Stride standing or sitting	Tuck the chin in and drop the head forward. Lift the chin and take the head backwards.
Stride standing or sitting	Look straight ahead and take the head sideways: ear towards shoulder, first to the right and then to the left.

Stride standing or sitting	Keep the chin in. Turn the head towards the right shoulder and then the left shoulder.
Stride standing or sitting	Tuck the chin in and drop the head forward. Keep the chin on the chest. Turn the head to the right and then left.

Do not circle the head round and round, as this can damage the cervical joints and cause pressure on the spinal nerves in this area.

Shoulder mobility

STARTING POSITION	EXERCISE
Stride standing or sitting	Pull the shoulder back and relax. Lift the shoulders up and down.
Stride standing or sitting	Circle the shoulders forward, upwards, backwards and down, then the other way.
Stride standing	Swing the arm forward above head and backwards.
Stride standing	Swing the arms sideways to cross above head then down to cross behind back.
Stride standing	Keep the elbows straight and rotate the arms medially and laterally (turn in and out).
Stride standing	Circle the arms alternately and then together (backwards).
Stride standing	Swing the arms alternately and then together (backwards).
Stride standing	Raise arms sideways to clap above head and then lower to clap at sides.
Stride standing	Raise arms sideways to clap above head and then lower to clap at sides.

Stride standing	Place right hand behind head and left arm behind back, trying to touch hands, then change.
Stride standing or sitting	Reach forward, keep arms at shoulder level. Cross the arms and clasp the hands. Lift arms above head and down behind head.
Yard stride standing	Bend elbows with palms facing forward. Drop the arms so that the palms face backwards. Rotate the arms up and down.

Combination of the above movements can be used and performed to music. Towels, bars and dumb bells can be used to add variety and interest.

Prone kneeling on elbows (not hands)	Rest chin on one hand. Take the other arm under the body and stretch down the outside of opposite leg. Take out and lift out to the side.

Trunk mobility

STARTING POSITION	EXERCISE
Stride standing, hands on thighs	Keep chin in. Curl the trunk forwards while sliding the hands down the thigh.
Stride standing, hands on buttocks	Extend the trunk backwards while sliding the hands down the buttocks.
Stride standing, hands to sides	Bend the trunk to the right and then to the left while sliding the hands down the sides.
Bend stride standing	Twist the trunk to the right and then to the left.
Reach stride standing	Twist the trunk to the right and then left.

Crook lying	Press lower back into floor. Bend alternate legs onto chest.
Crook lying	Bring both legs onto chest.
Crook lying	Bring both legs onto chest. Lift head and shoulders towards knees, clasping the knees with the hands.
Crook lying	Keep the shoulders against the floor. Tip both knees to the right and then to the left. Keep knees together.
Supine lying	Stretch right arm down right side and left arm down left side.
Prone kneeling with back flat	Arch the back upwards, pull in the tummy, lower back and hollow gently.
Prone kneeling with back flat	Bend right knee onto chest, arch back and kick out behind, repeat with left.
Prone kneeling	Stretch opposite arm and leg outwards and upwards. Repeat with other side.
Supine lying	Take right leg at right angles to the body. Lower the leg towards left floor, twisting the trunk gently. Repeat for other leg.
Prone lying	Lift opposite arm and leg upwards. Repeat.

Hip mobility exercises

STARTING POSITION	EXERCISE
Support standing	Raise one leg and swing forward and backwards. Keep the toes pointing forward, do not move the trunk and keep the hip forward. Repeat with other leg.

Support standing	Raise one leg sideways and swing sideways and back across the other leg. Keep the toe pointing forward and do not move the trunk. Repeat with the other leg.
Support standing	Raise one leg and circle around. Repeat with the other leg.
Prone kneeling	Bend knee up to chest and kick out and up. Repeat with the other leg.
Supine lying	Part legs and bring together.
Crook lying	Drop knees outwards and bring together.
Supine lying	Bend knees onto chest and straight into the air; keep at 90° to the body. Open and cross legs in scissor movement. Bend knees to chest, to lower.
Prone lying	Bend knees to right angles, slightly apart. Swing feet out sideways and inwards to cross legs.
Standing	Run on the spot, lifting knees higher and higher.
Standing	Star jumping – legs sideways.
Standing	Jumping legs, forward and backwards.

Knee mobility

STARTING POSITION	EXERCISE
High sitting on high chair or end of couch	Swing the legs up and down, from bend to straight knee.
Prone lying on a couch with feet over the end	Alternately bend knees, bringing heel to buttock and straighten.

Prone lying on a couch with feet over the end	Bend one knee, cross the other leg over back of leg. Now push with the back leg to increase the bend in the front leg. This is useful if there is limited range in the knee joint. Repeat with other leg.
Supine lying	Bend one knee onto chest. Kick out straight and lower. If bending is limited, grasp the knee with hands and pull into body. Repeat with the other leg. (DO NOT perform this exercise with both legs together.)
Supine lying	Bend knees onto chest and straighten into the air. Cycle the legs in the air.
Standing, hold onto wall bar with hands at shoulder height	Bend knees and hips down to the squatting position, hold and straighten. (*Caution:* do not take buttock below knees)

Use an exercise bike, and cycle with the saddle as low as possible.

Foot: Strengthening and mobilising

STARTING POSITION	EXERCISE
Sitting feet on floor	■ Push toes into floor (do not let them curl). ■ Raise toes away from floor. ■ Spread toes outwards and together. ■ Move big toes towards each other. ■ Pick up a pencil with the toes.

Sitting feet on floor with towel or strap lengthways under foot	Keep the heel firmly pressed onto towel, then use toes to pull and ruck the towel towards the heel.
Sitting feet on floor with towel or strap widthways under foot	Keep heel on ground and move towel to one side and then the other.
Sitting with hands over top of toes	Push down with hand and lift the toes up against the resistance.
Sitting with hands under the toes	Push up with the hand and push down with the toes against resistance.
Sitting one leg across the other at knee	Turn foot in and out.
Sitting one leg across the other at knee	Pull the foot up and down.
Sitting one leg across the other at knee	Circle the foot 10 times one way, and then the opposite way.
Long sitting	Turn feet inwards, press inner arches together.

- Walk around moving from heel, outer border to inner ball of foot.
- Walk in a straight line moving from heel, outer border to inner ball of foot.
- Walk around on toes.
- Walk around on heels.
- Walk normally.
- Skip or jog, changing direction.
- Hop on one leg then the other.
- Jumping forward, backwards, sideways.
- Jumping to stride and back, jump to walk and back, squat jump.

Warm up exercises

These exercises are performed at the beginning of an exercise class, training session or athletic performance. They bring the body slowly to a level which will enable the individual to perform at maximal potential, and also will reduce the risk of injury. The length of time spent on warm up will depend on environmental temperature; on cold days a longer warm up will be required.

The warm up should be long enough to produce a light sweating (approximately 10–15 minutes). This is a good indication that the body temperature has been raised sufficiently to begin the stretch programme.

Effects of warm up

A warm up should:

- raise the body temperature
- increase cardio-respiratory response
- increase blood flow to the muscles, and therefore increase oxygen and nutrient delivery
- increase muscle cell metabolism
- increase speed of nerve impulse transmission to the muscles
- increase the elasticity and extensibility of ligaments, tendons and muscles, thus reducing stiffness and risk of tear injuries
- raise hormonal response.

All the large muscle groups must be included in the warm up; ie, the muscles of the calf, the quadriceps, the hamstrings, the abdominals and the shoulder muscles. It is also important to include all the muscles used in the main scheme or performance. These may include the hip abductors and adductors, gluteus maximus, the pectorals, trapezius, back extensors, biceps and triceps.

Always begin with easy gentle exercises and progress to the more difficult.

Sample warm up exercises

(The starting position is standing.)

- Alternate heel raising
- Walking around the room
- Fast walking around the room
- Marching on the spot
- Marching around the room
- Knee bend and grasp with hands
- Skipping
- Cycling
- Jumping jacks (*caution:* do not adduct too far)
- Alternate leg swinging forward, backwards
- Alternate leg swinging sideways
- Hip circling
- Pelvic tilting forward and backwards
- Hip and trunk rotation clockwise and anticlockwise
- Trunk twisting to right and left
- Trunk side bends (*caution:* keep arms to sides)
- Shoulder shrugging
- Shoulder circling backwards and forwards
- Arm swinging across body
- Arm circling begin with small circles and increase range
- Elbow bend and extend with backward arm swing
- Alternate arm and trunk upward stretch
- Neck flexion, extension, side flexion and rotation.

Cool down exercises

These exercises are performed at the end of the class. They allow the body to return slowly to a state of balance (homeostasis). Cool down should include some stretching exercises of the main muscle groups to reduce soreness.

Do not stand still when performing cool down: walk, jog or perform exercises in sitting or lying positions. This is because the large blood vessels to the muscles of the legs are still dilated to meet the demand for more blood while exercising. The peripheral vessels are dilated to loose heat. While the leg muscles are contracting, they pump the blood back to the heart but when standing still, these muscles are not pumping and blood pools in the dilated blood vessels due to the pull of gravity. The heart is unable to maintain a sufficient blood supply to the brain, resulting in dizziness and fainting. Cool down should be performed for 10–15 minutes at the end of the class.

Sample cool down exercises:

- Skipping
- Jogging
- Walking
- Stepping
- Knee bends.

In sitting

- Neck flexion, extension, side flexion, rotation
- Shoulder shrugging
- Trunk rotation
- Trunk side flexion
- Trunk forward flexion
- Alternate knee bending grasp with hands and pull
- Latissimus dorsi and triceps stretch.

In lying

- Spinal rotation stretch
- Knee hug hamstring stretch
- Shoulder rotations
- Gastrocnemius stretch.

Prone lying

- Push up back extension
- Knee bend quadriceps stretch.

Long sitting

- Gastrocnemius stretch
- Hamstring stretch
- Spinal rotation stretch

(Descriptions of these exercises are found in Chapters 8 and 9.)

- End the class with deep breathing in the lying position.
- Get up slowly.

Breathing exercises

The thorax expands in three directions:

1 the sternum swings forwards
2 the ribs swing sideways and upwards
3 the diaphragm moves downwards.

Breathing exercises must maximise all these movements.

Technique

Sit in a comfortable position or lie down.

Apical expansion

Place the hands below each clavicle. Breathe in deeply through the nose, and concentrate the expansion beneath the hands. Feel the chest moving out towards the hands. Breathe out through the mouth and feel the chest sink back.

Costal expansion

Place the hands on the ribs just above the waist. Breathe in deeply through the nose and feel the ribs moving out sideways. Breathe out through the mouth and feel the ribs sink back.

Diaphragmatic expansion

Place the hands on the front, just on the midriff below the sternum. Breathe in through the nose and feel the abdomen expanding outwards. Breathe out through the mouth and pull the abdomen in.

Repeat each area three or four times. If you feel dizzy, take a break.

Potentially damaging exercises

There are a number of exercises that produce excessive stresses on vulnerable areas of the body (such as the neck, the lower back and the knees), and that may result in injury. They should not be performed by unfit people, nor included in general or group exercises where individual supervision and control is impossible. If they are performed by very fit athletes under controlled conditions, the risk of injury is greatly reduced. The ability to evaluate the safety and effectiveness of an exercise is an important part of an instructor's role. All exercise videos, exercise books and magazine articles must be carefully studied and each exercise analysed and checked for safety, as many of these hazardous exercises are included. New forms of routines require particular caution – the human body is designed to perform a certain finite number of movements through specific ranges, and the 'new' exercises must be versions of the old. Claims made for the results are often exaggerated; they are not realistic and achievable.

When assessing the safety and effectiveness of an exercise, it is useful to ask the following questions:

1 Will the exercise work the appropriate body part?
2 Will the exercise move the selected muscle and joint through the correct range?
3 Will the movement be controlled, free movement, and not forced or ballistic?
4 Is the exercise appropriate for this client's level of fitness?
5 Could the exercise over-stress the moving joints or other body parts, causing damage?
6 Is this the most suitable exercise for achieving the set goal?
7 Will the exercise or the starting position stress any of the following vulnerable areas?
    A the cervical region (the neck)
    B the lumbar region (the lower back)
    C the knees.

The cervical region 7 vertebrae

This is the region of greatest spinal mobility. The first two cervical vertebrae – atlas and axis, allow rotation of the head. The movement of the cervical region are:

- *Flexion:* drop the head forward, chin on chest.
- *Extension:* take the head backwards; hyper-extension takes it beyond extension to look at the ceiling.
- *Side flexion (lateral flexion):* drop the head sideways, ear towards shoulder.
- *Rotation:* turn the head to the right and left, looking toward the shoulder.
- *Circumduction:* a combination of the above.

Movements of the chin also affect the cervical region:

- protraction: pushing the chin forward.
- retraction: pulling the chin back and in.

Before commencing exercises for the cervical spine, select a stable starting position such as sitting or stride standing. If the client is very tense, the lying position can be used. Make sure the head is in a good position; ie, erect, ear lobes level, eyes looking straight ahead, shoulders relaxed.

Neck exercises

SAFE exercises

STARTING POSITION	EXERCISE
Sitting	Drop chin onto chest, return to upright position.
Sitting	Take right ear down towards right shoulder, then back, and left ear towards left shoulder.
Sitting	Turn the head to the right to look toward the right shoulder. Repeat on left.

(Instruction – keep the chin in and head up)

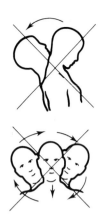

NOT recommended

Sitting	Hyperextension – dropping the head back to look at the ceiling.
Sitting	Head circling around on the shoulders.

These exercises produce excessive pressure and compression of the cervical discs. These may protrude into the intervertebral foramina resulting in pressure on, and damage to the nerves. This will cause pain, numbness, pins and needles over the shoulder and down the arm.

With age, the cervical region is susceptible to wear and tear, with erosion of the cartilage and bone. This may result in inflammation of surrounding structures, with pain and stiffness of the neck. These exercises will exacerbate this condition. The movements should only be performed by young, fit, well trained individuals. They should not be done in general exercise classes, by those over 30 years or by anyone suffering from headaches, neck pain or shoulder and arm pain, numbness or pins and needles.

The 'plough'

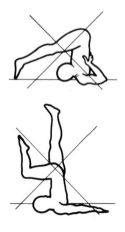

NOT recommended

STARTING POSITION	EXERCISE
Lying	Lift legs and lower back upwards to touch the floor behind the head with the toes.
Lying	Lift legs and hips off the floor and support with hands. Cycle or open/close legs in the air.

With both these exercises, the body weight is supported across the shoulders and neck. This imposes severe compression forces on the neck, which can cause damage to ligaments, bones, discs and nerves. This position also compresses the chest, thus reducing the working and efficiency of the heart and lungs.

The lumbar region 5 vertebrae

This is the lower back, and is a vulnerable area because it supports all the body weight before it is distributed to the pelvis. The movements of the lumbar region are:

- *Flexion:* bend forward.
- *Extension:* move the trunk backwards.
- *Limited side flexion:* bend to the side.
- *Negligible rotation:* turning the trunk right and left is negligible in the lumbar region (most trunk rotation occurs in the thoracic region).

The lumbar region is where most trunk flexion occurs and it is the *fulcrum* for this movement. (The *weight* is the upper trunk and the *weight arm* is the length of the trunk about the fulcrum. The *effort* is supplied by the back extensors and the *effort arm* is the distance of their insertion from the fulcrum. See Chapter 5 for a full explanation of levers in the body.) Considerable stress is placed on the lumbar spine during forward flexion and return to extension. The amount of stress is influenced by two factors:

1 The length of the weight arm and amount of weight.
2 The rotation of the pelvis which accompanies the movement.

The trunk extensors (erector spinae) and the antagonistic trunk flexors (the abdominals) must be strong and balanced to support the trunk and maintain the stability of the pelvis. Imbalance between these muscles alters pelvic tilt and imposes stresses on the lumbar spine:

- weakness of abdominals resulting in forward pelvic tilt and lordosis of lumbar spine.
- weakness of erector spinae resulting in backward pelvic tilt and flat back.

SAFE exercise

STARTING POSITION	EXERCISE
Stride standing, hands on legs (knees soft)	Slowly bend forward, sliding the hands down the legs, then return to upright position.

Particular care must be taken when coming up; always rotate the pelvis backwards first, and then extend the lumbar spine. Instruction on coming up should be: 'pull bottom in and straighten inch by inch from bottom of spine upwards'.

NOT recommended

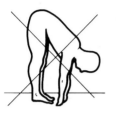

Stretch, stride standing	Bend forward to touch floor, and swing up.

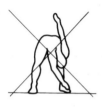

Stretch, stride standing	Bend to touch opposite foot and hand.

In these positions with the arms stretched above the head, the *weight arm* is lengthened and there is a far greater *load* in front of the *fulcrum* (lumbar spine). This increases the stress and compression on the discs, and damage can occur to ligaments, discs, cartilage or the bones. Punching the air with the hands in forward flexion imposes the same stress and is not recommended. Rotating the trunk to touch the opposite foot increases the compression forces still further.

Ballistic type bouncing at the end of the range of forward flexion to stretch the hamstrings must be avoided. This exerts excessive pressure on the lower back and may produce micro-tears and damage of the hamstrings. The hamstrings are not relaxed in this position but are contracting eccentrically, therefore stretching is ineffective and can cause damage.

SAFE exercise

STARTING POSITION	EXERCISE
Stride standing	Trunk side flexion to the right and left.

The same principle of leverage applies to this exercise and the exercise will be safe if the arms are kept down to the side keeping the weight arm as short as possible.

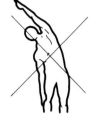

NOT recommended

Stride standing	Swing left arm into the air and side flex to the right. Come up. Swing right arm up and side flex to the left.

The arm is now stretched up into the air, increasing the length of the *weight arm*. The increased leverage imposes stresses on the lumbar joints and discs, causing damage. Ballistic bouncing at the end of the range will make the exercise even more hazardous.

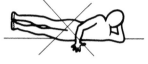

Side lying	Lift both legs upwards.

The trunk side flexors are straining to lift the legs. This stresses the lower back. Twisting of the trunk while straining to lift the legs, causes further damage.

Abdominal strengthening

SAFE exercise

STARTING POSITION	EXERCISE
Crook lying	Press small of back into floor. Tilt pelvis backwards and pull in the abdominals.
Crook lying, hands across chest	Curl up head towards knees.

This exercise can be safely progressed by moving the arm position, thus lengthening the weight arm; eg, hands on shoulders, hands beside head, hands stretched above head. It can be progressed further by holding a weight across the chest. (Do not clasp the hands behind the head as this can stress and damage the neck. Place hands at sides of the head over the ears.)

NOT recommended

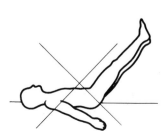

Lying	Double leg raising.

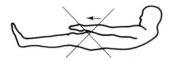

Lying   Straight back, sit ups.

Both these exercises impose stress and can cause many problems. They are not effective in strengthening the abdominal muscles, which can be seen by analysing the movement:

Moving joint: hip joint.
Direction of movement: flexion coming up, extension going down.
Prime movers: psoas – hip flexor.
Type of muscle work: coming up – psoas concentric, going down – psoas, eccentric.

■ Psoas is a short muscle passing from the lumbar vertebrae to the lesser trochanter of the femur. It works with iliacus, and both muscles may be named 'ilio psoas'. As psoas lifts the legs or the trunk, it pulls on its origin on the lumbar spine, imposing stresses and strains in this region. Psoas is working at tremendous mechanical disadvantage, as it is made to lift a long weight arm multiplied by the weight of the legs. The back arches and strain is felt in the lumbar spine.

■ With this exercise, psoas becomes stronger and tighter. This is undesirable because a tight psoas pulls and tilts the pelvis forwards, resulting in lordosis (due to muscle imbalance).

■ The abdominal muscles will be working statically in outer range, in an attempt to keep the pelvis level. This type of muscle work is extremely difficult to maintain and can only be done by very strong muscles; weaker muscles will be strained.

■ Static work of the abdominals increases intra-abdominal pressure which will push on the pelvic organs and stretch pelvic floor. The muscles of the pelvic floor may already be weakened in post natal women and older age groups.

Back strengthening exercises

SAFE exercise

STARTING POSITION	EXERCISE
Prone lying	Alternate single leg raising.
Prone lying	Alternate arm raising.
Prone lying	Opposite arm and leg raising.

NOT recommended

Prone lying	Double leg raising.
Prone lying	Double leg, arm and trunk raising.
Prone lying	Trunk extension, touching feet with hands.

Raising both legs (or worse, raising both legs and arms) imposes severe compression and stress on the lumbar spine.

Gluteal strengthening

SAFE exercise

STARTING POSITION	EXERCISE
Prone lying	Raise alternate legs off the floor and lower (keep hips in contact with the floor and lift upwards 15° from floor).

Prone kneeling	Straighten alternate leg backwards. Lift to just 15° from horizontal; lower.

NOT recommended

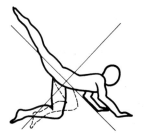

Prone kneeling	Bend knee onto chest and kick out behind.

Raising the leg backwards beyond 15° to the horizontal can stress the lumbar spine. The exercise uses the hip flexor (ilio psoas) to bend the knee towards the chest (this does not usually require strengthening). This exercise is frequently performed in a swinging manner when the movement is not controlled and likely to cause damage.

The knee joint

The stability of the knee is maintained by:

- several strong ligaments (the medial and lateral ligaments and the cruciate ligaments)
- powerful muscles (the quadriceps and hamstrings)
- the fascia of the thigh (fascia lata).

The movements of the knee are:

1 *Flexion:* bending the knee
2 *Extension:* straightening the knee

A slight amount of rotation is possible in flexion.

Hamstring stretch (hurdler's stretch)

SAFE exercise

STARTING POSITION	EXERCISE
Long sitting	Bend right knee and rotate hip outwards. Drop knee onto floor and place foot against left thigh. Place hands on either side of left leg and gently slide hands down left leg forwards. Repeat on opposite side.

NOT recommended

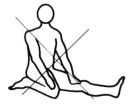

Long sitting	Bend right knee, turn leg backwards, slide hands along left leg to touch toes.

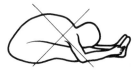

Long sitting	Forward flexion, bring head down to knees.

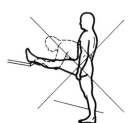

The position of the flexed knee backwards stresses the medial ligaments of the knee. This method also stresses the lower back. The forward hurdler's stretch also stresses the back.

Standing	Right leg at right angles resting on chair, bend forward sliding hands down left leg.

Squatting

SAFE exercise

STARTING POSITION	EXERCISE
Standing or walk standing	Bend knees until they are at 90°. Do not allow buttocks to go below the knees.

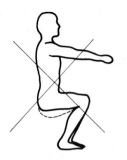

NOT recommended

Standing or walk standing	Bend or squat beyond 90°.
Squatting	Jumping and stretching leg out to side.

Bending the knees beyond 90° while supporting body weight can impose severe stress on the knee joint.

Heel sitting

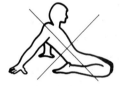

This position should be avoided by all except the young and very fit clients as it stresses and can damage the knee joint. The body weight is opening up and adding pressure to the knee joint, which can damage the cartilage and strain ligaments.

Kneeling and modifications of kneeling should not be used as a starting position for the older client, or for anyone with knee pain.

Damaging exercises to avoid

- Double leg raising or sit ups with straight legs.
- Hurdle stretch, both standing and long sitting.
- Pliés.
- Deep squats
- Forward flexion where the trunk is at 90° to legs.
- legs in air resting on head and shoulders ('the plough').
- Head circling.
- Head hyper extension.
- Very wide jumping jacks with knees opening wider than toes; keep knees in line with toes.
- Any ballistics, ie, bouncing at the end of range such as toe touching, side bending, trunk twisting.

- Heel sitting, up to kneeling should only be performed by the young and athletic, ie, those with strong quadriceps. It should not be performed by anyone with knee problems nor over 40 years of age. The same applies to exercises using kneeling as a starting position.
- Back hyper extension.

Questions

1 List the five basic starting positions.
2 Explain the following terms:
  A prone lying
  B crook sitting
  C stride standing
3 Draw diagrams to illustrate the following arm positions:
  A wing standing
  B across bend standing
  C yard standing
4 Give two exercises to improve mobility in each of the following joints:
  A shoulder joint
  B hip joint
  C knee joint.
5 List six effects of warm up exercises.
6 List six examples of warm up activities.
7 Explain why the client should not stand still when performing cool down exercises.
8 Give the reason for including some stretch exercises in the cool down routine.
9 Describe the three directions of thoracic expansion during deep breathing.
10 Describe where the hands should be placed when teaching diaphragmatic expansion.
11 Name the three most vulnerable areas to stress, when performing exercises.
12 Describe the symptoms of damage to the cervical region.
13 Explain why the 'plough' is not a recommended exercise.
14 Explain in detail, why 'double leg raising' or 'straight back sit ups' should *not* be given as an exercise to strengthen the abdominal muscles.
15 Explain why 'heel sitting' should not be used as a starting position.

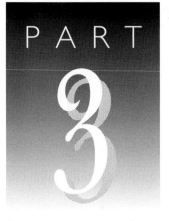
Teaching Exercises

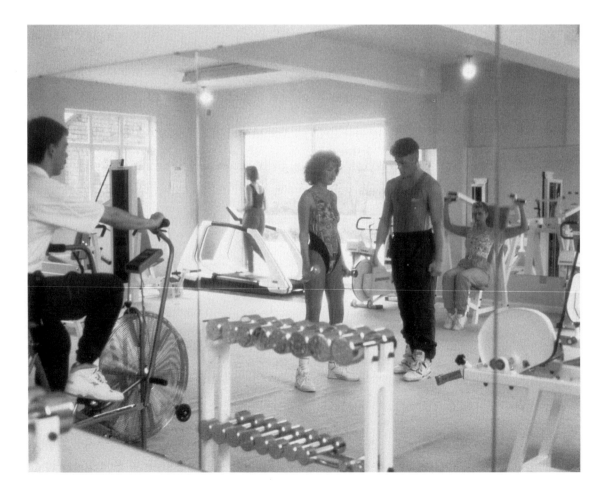

CHAPTER 13

The Acquisition of Skill

The teaching of exercises or the training for a specific activity requires the passing of 'knowledge of the skill' from the instructor to the learner/client. Throughout the training period the learner will be modifying his or her actions or behaviour while mastering the new skill. Learning a new skill is a very complex process.

Skill

Skilled movement is balanced, co-ordinated, graceful and precise, with accurate timing and overall rhythmic flow. There is no wastage of energy. The essential features of skilled performance are:

- accuracy of timing
- anticipation of movement
- economy of effort
- grace and precision of movement
- overall flow of the movement.

Skill improves as a result of practice and experience. A skill is goal directed; the learner must be aware of the desired end result and how to achieve it. Constant repetition of patterns of movement must be practised until they are registered in the brain and can eventually be performed automatically. Muscle strength, flexibility and co-ordination contribute to skilled performance, and repetition and practice is essential to achieve high standards. One method of learning an activity and maximise skill, is to break it down into small chunks or parts. Each part should be practised until a satisfactory standard is achieved. The sequence of movements is then linked, and the complete activity is practised, until all errors are eliminated and the performance is automatic. However, some performers will prefer to practise the whole sequence.

Learning new skills

The mastery of skills is a continuing process from birth to death; mastery of low level skills will prepare the way for learning skills at a higher level.

The high level skills required by athletes, gymnasts, etc, must be learned and continually practised to achieve peak performance. Skilled performance will involve the efficient use of physiological and psychological processes. It requires the use of both receptor and effector responses; ie, effective co-ordination between mind and muscle. There are very many theories related to the learning of motor skills, and their study is not within the scope of this book.

However, the two main groups are the *behaviourist* and the *cognitive* theorists:

1 The behaviourists believe that learning is the process of establishing bonds between stimuli and responses. The provision of a stimulus initiates a response: S–R bonding. The more frequently the S–R bond occurs, the more likely it is to be established. This bonding is strengthened if the learner gains satisfaction and reward.
2 The cognitive theorists emphasise the thought processes involved in learning:
   A understanding what is required and selecting the most appropriate methods of achieving the goal
   B using information received to correct errors and perfect performance.

Stages of learning

Paul Fitts, an American psychologist, proposed that the learner must pass through three overlapping phases when learning new skills:

1 *The cognitive phase:* During this phase, cognitive and

perceptual processes tend to dominate as the learner requires knowledge of the skill. The learner analyses the tasks and tries to understand what to do and how to do it. During this phase a large number of errors are made. The learner realises when an error has been made, but is unsure of how to correct it. At this stage, demonstration, cues and correction must be given frequently during the practice. Common errors must be pointed out so that they may be recognised and rectified.

2 *The associative phase:* The emphasis now changes to the psychomotor component of the skill; this phase is concerned with practising the new skill. As a result of practise, errors are gradually eliminated. Correct patterns are established, co-ordination and rhythm improve, errors are still made but are more easily recognised and corrected with minimal prompting.

3 *The autonomous phase:* Skills are now performed automatically and require little conscious control. The performance is efficient and consistent, errors have largely been eliminated or can be quickly corrected without prompting. Speed and accuracy are increased and the effects of stress reduced.

Throughout these phases of learning, the instructor must impart knowledge of how the skill is to be performed.

The cognitive phase is probably the most important phase when learning a new skill such as a movement or exercise. Any misunderstanding or misinterpretation at this stage will affect the ultimate performance. The objectives must be outlined, each part of the movement accurately and clearly explained and the criteria of evaluation emphasised:

- *Visual* guidance gives the learner a clear picture of what is required at all stages of the performance; the activity is demonstrated in its entirety at the correct rhythm and speed.
- *Verbal* guidance is also given through explanation, description, and corrective cues.
- *Manual* guidance may be given by physically moving a limb or turning the body into the correct position.

The learner will receive stimuli via the organs of sight and sound and touch, and these pass to the brain to be organised and retained. The demonstration must be one of excellence against which the learner can measure his own performance. Each component part of the movement may then be broken down into more manageable chunks and performed slowly, with verbal cues given to reinforce the visual. The criteria (conditions of the desired performance) are emphasised during this phase.

In the associative phase, practice is the essence. As a result of practice, a constant stream of stimuli will pass up to the brain where they will be organised and analysed. Some will be disregarded in favour of others. In response, impulses will flow from the brain to the muscles, stimulating their contraction. The brain registers patterns rather than individual movements, and the establishment of correct patterns will result in accurate skilled performance. With continued practice, guidance through corrective cues and feedback, the learner will refine the performance, selecting the correct effective actions and disregarding the inaccurate and ineffective.

In the autonomous phase, the learning is consolidated and the skill will be performed automatically. The learner will now be free to consider and practise the finer points in pursuit of excellence.

Motivation

Motivation is the drive within an individual to succeed. A high level of motivation will result in increased effort and the determination to improve performance. Motivation varies among individuals and personality types. Previous experiences of success and failure and many other factors will influence motivation. These factors may be intrinsic or extrinsic:

- *Intrinsic* factors come from within the individual, eg, feelings of well-being, happiness, pleasure, achievement, recognition, personal growth, satisfaction.
- *Extrinsic* factors come from external sources, eg, gaining status, awards, badges, financial gain.

Research indicates that intrinsic factors are the more important and produce better, longer lasting results. The good instructor, teacher or coach is able to encourage intrinsic factors and stimulate the student's motivation. The instructor can ensure that the class is well organised and administered, and that the teaching style is enthusiastic, positive, concerned, caring, pleasant, knowledgeable and safe. A high level of expertise should be demonstrated at all times, both in theoretical knowledge and practical demonstration.

It is the teacher's responsibility to prevent or guard against any demotivating factors such as poor facilities, unpleasant surroundings, lack of organisation, poor safety and hygiene conditions; showing lack of interest and/or expertise, creating feelings of dissatisfaction, failure, embarrassment; setting unrealistic goals that are not achievable.

Feedback

Giving guidance and continuous feedback throughout the session will enhance motivation. Feedback is essential as it ensures the learner is aware of a correct or incorrect performance. Errors must be eliminated as early as possible to ensure that they are not reinforced.

Millar, an American psychologist, distinguishes between two forms of feedback:

1 *Action feedback* provides knowledge of current progress; actions are corrected as they are performed. The instructor must therefore provide cues during performance of the exercise. Appropriate cues include: 'eyes front', 'hold the head up', 'shoulders down', 'knees higher', 'do not stretch too far', 'do not lift too high'.
2 *Learning feedback* provides information which enables the student to improve next time. As she sees the result of an action, she tries to improve it on the next attempt. Appropriate cues are: 'Take the arm back further', 'Did you keep the back straight?', 'Well done but keep that tummy in', 'Well done but watch that you roll the pelvis backwards before you come up', 'I obviously didn't explain that exercise clearly', explain again and demonstrate with 'Watch me again'. In this way members can correct their performance and will move quickly into the autonomous phase.

Many corrective statements and cues will be required for new members of a class or when learning a new exercise, but as the skill is mastered fewer cues are needed. Positive value statements such as 'good', 'that's better', 'well done', 'great'. These will encourage members and increase motivation. It is always important to encourage and never to put anyone down, draw attention to poor performance or embarrass the learner. In a class, if only one or two members are not performing correctly, give a general corrective statement, catch their eye and say 'watch me', or explain the correction quietly and privately at the end of the class.

Planning exercise classes

Exercise classes can be designed to improve one or many of the components of fitness discussed in Chapter 7. Different forms of exercise must be selected to overload the appropriate systems depending on the desired outcomes of the group. Exercise classes in general are designed to improve the overall fitness of large numbers of people rather than the specific fitness of elite athletes. However, they are also used to improve the specific fitness required for particular sporting activities, eg, team training for soccer, rugby, basketball; group exercise prior to skiing, or water sport holidays etc. Although classes may offer different types of exercise, there are certain basic principles that apply to them all.

When dealing with mixed groups, it is very important to recognise and allow for individual differences within a group, ie, different intellectual levels, fitness levels, body shapes, health differences, previous experiences, life styles, age ranges and motivation. It is desirable but not always possible to organise classes so that there is parity within the group, eg, similar fitness levels, similar age groups, similar desired outcomes, etc. Alternatively classes may be structured to provide a suitable level for beginners, intermediate and advanced learners. Others may be structured according to age, eg, under 30's, over 30's, over 50's.

The principles of exercise (discussed in previous chapters) must be considered when planning exercise classes; these are:

■ Specificity
■ Training threshold
■ Overload
■ Progression
■ Intensity
■ Duration
■ Frequency

- Reversibility
- Long- and short-term planning: plan long-term objectives and time span (macrocycle); plan blocks for the systems to be trained (mesocycle); plan the activities for each class (microcycle).

Setting objectives or goals

This is the first step and a very important part of planning for group or individual exercises. Specific objectives must be set according to the aspirations and the desired outcomes of the individuals. The objectives must be realistic and attainable within a set timescale; they must be fully discussed and agreed by all concerned. The setting of long-term goals and short-term goals which are continually monitored through regular assessment will increase motivation. The objectives will depend on which components require improving; for example, the objectives may be to:

- increase cardio-respiratory fitness (aerobic work)
- improve muscle strength (resistance training)
- improve flexibility (stretch exercises)
- reduce fatty deposits (aerobic work)
- improve body shape (aerobic and resistance work)
- improve posture (stretch for tight muscles, strengthening for weak muscles)
- correct figure faults (as above)
- improve speed and skill
- improve general fitness

General fitness classes will include the components commonly referred to as the three **Ss**:

- **Stamina** – cardiovascular fitness (aerobic fitness).
- **Strength** – muscle strength.
- **Suppleness** – flexibility.

Lesson plans for each session should be prepared, as a record of work and to show progression. Each lesson plan should include:

- the objectives
- the sequence of activities ie, discussion, warm up/stretch, main conditioning, cool down.
- the time for each sequence
- the music (if used)

■ the equipment necessary
■ any comments or notes.

The sequence of activities

There will be four main phases to consider: discussion, warm up/stretch, main conditioning, cool down.

Discussion

It is important to begin each class with an introduction and an explanation of the planned activities. Members should be encouraged to ask questions and have problems clarified. This will take 5–10 minutes.

Warm up/stretch

This is an extremely important part of any exercise scheme and must be performed by all members of the class before moving into the main core or conditioning phase. Individuals who arrive late must perform the warm up routine before joining the class.

The warm up phase brings the body systems slowly to a level that will enable the individual to perform at maximal potential and reduce the risk of injury. The heart rate will gradually increase, breathing will become faster and deeper, the circulation will increase and more oxygen and nutrients will be delivered to the muscles; there will be a rise in body temperature, muscle cellular metabolism will increase, as will muscle flexibility and extensibility. Warm up should include all the large muscle groups, begin easily and gently, then gradually increase in intensity. This will take 10–15 minutes (see page 212 for further detail).

The stretch phase must follow the initial warm up. This moves the muscles and joints through their full range of movement. Normal daily activities require mainly mid-range movements, and muscles and joints rarely work in outer range. However, exercises may require full or outer range movements; it is therefore important to prepare the muscles and work them in outer range to prevent injury and maximise performance. The main muscles that require stretching are the calf, the hamstrings, the hip flexors, the adductors, the extensors of the back, latissimus dorsi, the pectorals. This will take 5–10 minutes (see page 159 for further detail).

The timing of the warm up/stretch routine will vary depending on the age or fitness level of the group and the temperature in the exercise room. The session should be longer for the mature client and the unfit, and in a cool environment.

The main core/conditioning phase

This is the most important phase of the class. The exercises selected will be specific to the set objectives; ie, to improve cardio vascular endurance, aerobic exercises will be planned, whereas to improve strength, resisted exercises must be planned. Consideration must be given to the principles of overload, intensity, duration and frequency. The exercises should begin gently, build up gradually to peak intensity and then ease off. This phase will last for 20–30 minutes.

Cool down

Exercising should never stop abruptly but taper off gradually. This phase enables the body to return slowly to a balanced state. Rhythmical movements which decrease in intensity must be performed so that the regular pumping action of the muscles maintains blood flow and flushes out lactic waste. Stretching exercises should be included to reduce muscle soreness. Cool down should end with deep breathing and relaxation in lying. This phase will take 7–10 minutes (see page 213 for further detail).

The preparation of a class

It is essential to prepare the environment where learning is to take place:

- Prepare the room before members arrive.
- Ensure that the lighting and ventilation are adequate. The room should be warm but not hot. Exercising in a hot environment can lead to heat exhaustion and dehydration.
- Check that the floor is firm, clean and smooth.
- Ensure that each person has sufficient space; 3–5 square feet per person is recommended, depending on the exercise. Less movement will require less space.
- Locate the first aid box and note all the exits.

- Check that the area is clear of equipment, apparatus or anything that may be a safety hazard.
- Select all required equipment or apparatus, and check that it is in good working order (so that the sequence of the class is not broken and learning disrupted).
- Arrange all equipment neatly at one end of the room, well away from the working area.
- Select the music tapes or records and stack them in order of use.
- Check that the music centre or player is working and that the sound is of good quality.
- Provide a large clock with a second hand to be used when monitoring heart rate.
- Ensure that there is water available at all times and encourage members to drink at regular intervals.
- Shower and change into appropriate clothes. Remember that you set the standard for the class: you should wear clean, unrestricting, absorbent, smart clothing and suitable footwear (see Chapter 1).
- Tie hair back and remove jewellery.

When members arrive:

- Greet members warmly, use their names where possible, make eye contact to show each member that they are recognised.
- Make a point of greeting and speaking to new members.
- Carry out a consultation/assessment of each new member. Check for any contra-indications and ensure that they have read the instructions (see Chapter 14) and signed the consent form.
- Check that members are wearing suitable, unrestricting clothing. Well cushioned shoes which provide adequate support, flexibility and cushioning must be worn.
- Check that hair is tied back and jewellery is removed.

During the class

- Begin the class on time!
- Step confidently in front of the class, speak clearly and make sure that those at the back can hear. Use the voice to good effect, change the tone to govern speed, rhythm, intensity and effort.
- Remember that you are the role model for the class, so develop a friendly, enthusiastic and positive approach.

Good posture, an alert and efficient manner will set the tone of the class. Do not fidget or develop irritating mannerisms such as tossing hair, or rubbing the leg.

- When demonstrating exercise, ensure that the performance is as accurate and perfect as possible. Poor demonstration means poor performance and ineffective exercise, which may also impose stresses on the body and cause strain and injury.
- Explain: the reasons for and the effects of each exercise; the health and benefits of exercise (see Chapter 2).
- Following demonstration, give clear simple commands and give corrective cues, particularly in the early stages.
- Break down complicated exercise into manageable 'chunks'. Teach one part at a time until each is well executed, and then perform together as a whole.
- Give encouragement to enhance motivation, ie, 'well done', 'that's good', 'much better', 'a great effort' etc.
- Take time to explain and teach new exercises.
- Stress that each individual must work at her own pace; no one should exceed the maximum heart rate. New members should work at 60% of MHR working up to 80% (see Chapter 8).
- Stop exercising if there are signs of stress such as:
  - A profuse sweating
  - B breathlessness
  - C tightness in the chest
  - D pain in the chest or arms
  - E pain in back or any joints
  - F faintness or dizziness
  - G headache
  - H nausea
  - I heart rate above maximum.
- Explain the importance of maintaining good posture; give advice on protecting the back, neck and knees. Instruct clients on how to get down and up off the floor:
  - A Going down: 'Down on hands and knees, roll onto side and then onto the back.'
  - B Coming up: 'Roll onto side, then onto hands and knees, then stand up.'
- Explain the importance of breathing normally and not holding the breath; breathe in before effort or on release and breathe out on effort, when you perform the exercise.
- Explain and give reasons for the importance of warm up (see page 212). Emphasise that even if members turn up late, they must not join the class until they have

completed the 10 minute warm up. They must do this at the edge or back of the class and then join in the other exercises. Explain the importance of stretch and the associated hazards. See Chapter 9.

■ Explain the importance of cool down, to allow the body to return slowly to the balanced state. Explain why cool down exercises should be performed in lying or while continuously moving around.

Types of aerobic classes

The American College of Sports Medicine defines aerobic activity as activity 'requiring continuous, rhythmic use of large muscle groups at 60–90% of the maximum heart rate and 50–85% of maximum oxygen uptake for 20–60 minutes, at least 3 times per week'. The main effects of aerobic exercises are:

■ an increase in cardio-respiratory fitness
■ a reduction in fatty deposits with resultant weight loss
■ an increase in muscular endurance
■ maintaining bone mass.

There are various activities designed to keep the body in continuous rhythmic motion and the list is continually growing. We have high, moderate, low impact, step, dance, water aerobics, etc.

High impact aerobics where both feet leave the ground are no longer recommended as they place members at risk of injury due to continuous jarring. Low impact where one foot always stays in contact with the ground and knees are slightly bent, is safer. Moderate impact will include some high impact but mainly low impact work. It is more desirable to concentrate on the duration and intensity rather than on impact.

■ Duration is increased by greater repetitions.
■ Intensity is increased by using longer and higher steps; move from jogging to marching to high stepping. Arm positions can change from waist or sides, to shoulder level, to above head; light ankle and wrist weights can be used. Fitter members can exaggerate movements taking bigger steps and travelling more.

Energy expenditure will depend on the intensity and

duration of the exercises: the higher, faster and longer the movements, the greater will be the energy expenditure.

As with all classes it is important to begin gradually. This allows the body to adapt to increased demand.

- The heart must adapt to maintain adequate blood supply to the working muscles.
- Blood flow will be diverted from the organs to the muscles.
- The respiratory rate must increase gradually to ensure adequate ventilation. Too rapid an increase in breathing will result in hyper ventilation and side cramps.

Plan the class as outlined in page 234. There are many different formats to choose from which depend on the sequencing of the exercises; eg, single peak, reverse peak, multi-peak, continuous peak. They all produce an aerobic effect and must include warm up, stretch, main core exercises and cool down. Relaxation and breathing may also be included if appropriate.

Selecting music

Selecting music is an important part of the planning. The music will set the 'mood' of the class; it provides timing for the exercises and keeps the class working together. It helps to provide interest, fun and enjoyment, and also increases motivation. When selecting music, consider the age range and lifestyle of the clients where possible; eg, the younger clients will enjoy contemporary pop music, while older clients may prefer 1960s music, big bands, folk, Country and Western, gospel or square dance music. Consider also the time of year, eg, Christmas music, summer songs etc. If the class is mixed, use a variety of music. Ask class members if they have favourite records or tapes that they would like to use. Use good quality equipment, and when taping music, vary the volume to suit the activity.

The choreography (the planning of the movements and sequences of music) must be done well in advance. This is difficult at first but becomes easier with practice. Watch exercise videos: see how the steps match the beat of the music. Watch modern dance and ballet: observe how foot, trunk and arm movements fit the music.

Study aerobic exercise books for different types of exercises or combination. Analyse and evaluate – are the exercises safe? are they appropriate? do they use the required muscles?

Planning exercises to music

- List all the foot and leg movements that you may wish to include in the class.
- List all the arm movements that may be performed on their own or to accompany the leg movements; see Table 13.1.

Table 13.1 Leg and arm movements

Leg movement	Arm movement
Heel raise	Hands on waist (wing)
Jog	Hands on shoulders (bend)
March	Arms out to side or front
High knee march	Arms on head
Walk	Arms reach up
Steps forward, back, side	Alternate reach up
Step touches	Alternate reaches sideways
Step kick	Swinging forward and back
Step knee lift	Sideways clap
Step knee lift and kick	Shoulder shrugging
Plié (caution)	Shoulder circling
Grapevine (cross one leg in front or behind the other)	Air punching forwards and upwards
Hopscotch	Across body swing
Rabbit hops	

List floor and stretch exercises in the same way.

Listen carefully to each piece of music and note:

1 The *rhythm*: this is the regular pattern of sound which will dictate the style of the exercise routine.
2 The *beat*: these are the pulsations of music. The beat is very important as the steps or movements are selected to accompany each beat.
3 The timing or number of beats in each bar. 3/4 time is used for the waltz, 2/4 or 4/4 time for marching and the polka. 2/4 and 4/4 time are best for class work. Waltz time can be used for stretching.
4 The *tempo*: the rate at which the music is played.

The American Aerobics Dance and Exercise book suggests that:

- slow tempos of 100–120 beats per minute (BPM) are suitable for warm up and cool down
- under 100 BPM for stretch and floor exercises
- faster tempos of 130–160 used for aerobics and dance.

The Fitness Leaders Handbook suggests:

- Warm up: 128–138 BPM
- Jump: 148–156
- Run: 160–174
- Low impact aerobics: 134–144
- Floor: 100–126
- Cool down: 110 and below.

Having listened to the music, select from the list of exercises suitable movements and patterns to fit the music. Practise these thoroughly on your own, and record each movement and series of movements (movements or patterns are usually repeated 4–6 times). Cue for good posture, breathing, accurate steps and movements throughout.

Questions

1 List the features that contribute to skilled performance.
2 Describe the three phases which the learner must pass through when learning new skills.
3 Explain the difference between the following types of guidance given to a learner of new skills:
   A Visual
   B Verbal
   C Manual
4 List six intrinsic factors which enhance motivation.
5 Explain why it is important to provide 'Feedback' during the learning process.
6 List the features which should be included in a lesson plan.
7 Describe how you would prepare the room prior to taking an exercise class.
8 List the signs which may indicate that the exerciser is stressed and should stop exercising.

CHAPTER 14

Planning and Assessment

Preparing a programme for a client is an extremely important task. It must ensure that the needs and desired outcomes/goals of the client are understood, and that they are realistic and achievable within the allocated time span. If the client's objectives are unrealistic, they must be discussed, and more realistic goals suggested and agreed. Goals should be dictated by the client, and agreed by the therapist; specific training routines and exercise are then planned to achieve the set objectives. The therapist and client must agree times and forms of assessment to measure progress. All data must be carefully recorded throughout the programme.

Planning

Planning can be broken down into the following steps:

1 Getting to know the client.
2 Assess fitness.
3 Write the programme.
4 Record of progress.

Getting to know the client

This is a very important step and sufficient time must be allowed to ensure a thorough consultation; it should not be hurried. Sit down with the client and make him/her comfortable – show that you are interested and supportive. Establish the following facts:

■ Why does the client want to improve fitness? What are the client's desired outcomes/goals? Try to establish a specific goal; eg 'I want to lose weight for my wedding in six months' time'. Specific goals increase motivation and the client is more likely to stay the course because of the specific time scale. Vague goals such as 'My husband said that I should lose weight' are unlikely to produce the same drive, and the likelihood of giving up is increased.

- Establish the client's lifestyle and level of activities (eg, highly active, moderate or inactive). How long has the client been inactive?
- What activities does the client like or dislike?
- Does the client exercise regularly? If so, what type of exercise, for how long and how often?
- Has the client exercised regularly in the past? How long ago did she exercise? Were goals achieved? What were the reasons for stopping?
- Is the client healthy, or are there any problems? Do these need medical referral?
- Check for contra-indications to exercise (see page 11).
- What are the client's nutritional habits? Is advice required?
- Does the client fully understand and agree with the set objectives and the methods by which they will be achieved?
- How much time can the client devote to the exercise?
- Is the client prepared to practise some exercises at home if required?
- Complete a **consultation form** and a **consent form** which must be signed by the client.

Assess fitness

Fitness assessment can vary, from sophisticated tests carried out under laboratory conditions, to simple tests described later in this chapter. The results of these tests must be recorded and used to measure progress or compare with standard 'norms'.

Write the programme

1 Write down the long-term objectives and the available time span.
2 Write down the short-term objectives (eg, gains every month) and how improvement is assessed.

3 Write down a plan for each lesson:

First of all decide on the type of exercises to be used. This will depend on the physiological systems to be trained eg, muscle strength, muscle endurance, cardio respiratory endurance etc.; on the likes and dislikes of the client; on availability of equipment and the working area.

Then consider and apply the principles of exercises; see pages 116 for a full explanation of the following terms:

- Overload
- Progression
- Specificity
- Regression
- Intensity
- Duration
- Frequency.

The training of athletes and sportspeople tends to fall into distinct seasons or periods. The programme is broken up to allow for different types of training within these periods, so that fitness is built up gradually, to peak at the event. This is referred to as a *periodised* training programme. Trainers divide the programme into cycles called megacycles, macrocycles, mesocycles and microcycles:

- Megacycle – a long period where the long-term goal may be winning a major championship.
- Macrocycle – a shorter period where the goal may be an intermediate championship.
- Mesocycle – monthly or set blocks of training; different forms of training are planned for each block, eg, strength, endurance, speed, flexibility.
- Microcycle – weekly training routines which are planned and adjusted to achieve the outcome identified in the mesocycle.

Record of progress

Progress must be recorded throughout the programme and discussed with the client, as this increases motivation. If the client can see an improvement, s/he is more likely to continue with the programme. With weight lifting for strength, progression is obvious because heavier weights are lifted, but for endurance, the pulse rate or VO_2 must be recorded; for body composition, fat calliper measurement or body measurement gives feedback.

Assessment

The assessment of a client prior to exercise has developed considerably over the last few years. In addition to information regarding health, medical history, measurements of height, weight, fat distribution and muscle tone, it is now desirable to assess fitness by measuring pulse rate, blood pressure, lung capacity, muscle strength, muscle endurance, flexibility and body composition. Simple tests can be carried out in the gym or fitness centre, and are described below.

Accurate assessment is important as it:

- provides information on past and present state of health. This will highlight any contra-indications or any conditions where caution is necessary.
- provides information on lifestyle, activities, athleticism and client motivation.
- establishes the figure type, ie, endomorph, ectomorph or mesomorph, which facilitates the planning and setting of realistic, achievable goals.
- identifies postural problems and muscle imbalance so that specific strategies to restore balance can be planned.
- establishes the current level of fitness, which provides a starting point for the exercise programmes.
- provides the information necessary for setting objectives and the planning of safe, effective exercise which will not place the client at risk.
- provides a record of data and the starting point from which future improvement can be measured.
- provides motivation for improvement.

Preparation of the client prior to fitness assessment

Advise the client:

- to wear comfortable loose fitting clothes
- not to eat for two to three hours before the test
- not to smoke before or during the test
- not to drink tea or coffee before the test

CONSENT FORM

Personal details:

Name   Date of birth
Address   Tel no: home
                                                          work

Occupation

Doctor's name   Surgery tel no.:
Doctor's address

Medical history:
Past health problems

Present state of health

Medication

Leisure activities:
Exercise or activity likes and dislikes

Date of previous training or exercise programme

Type of exercise/training undertaken

Present objectives:

Recommended exercise plan:

Consent:
I agree to take part in the assessment and in the exercise programme which has been recommended,
explained and discussed with me. I fully understand my commitment and what is required of me. I
have read the list of guidelines for exercises and the list of contra-indications and have discussed
these with the instructor. I know of no reason why I should not undertake the recommended exercise
programme.
I am aware that I must stop exercising immediately and must inform the instructor if I experience
any pain, discomfort or severe breathlessness during the programme. I understand that regular
practice is required to achieve the set goals but that I am free to withdraw from the programme
at any time.
I undertake to inform my instructor if there is any change in my medical condition during the
course of the programme and I will obtain my doctor's consent to continue if necessary.

Name of client:
Signature of client:
Signature of witness:
Date:

Figure 14.1   *A sample consent form*

- to empty the bladder before the test
- to avoid other exercises before the test
- to concentrate fully on the test
- to say immediately if they do not understand the instructions and what is required of them.

POINTS TO CONSIDER

The therapist should make sure that the tests are:

- accurately performed
- standardised and consistent
- valid; do they test what they claim to test?
- reliable; each test should be carried out by the same person, at the same time of day and under the same conditions.

Height measurement

Instruct the client to:

- stand in bare feet
- put feet together
- back against measure
- stand straight and look directly ahead.

Bring measure bar to just touch the head, read the measurement, record on client's card and inform the client.

Weight measurement

Instruct the client to:

- wear minimum clothing (record this to ensure that the same clothing is worn each time weight is taken)
- stand in bare feet
- stand in the centre of the weighing machine
- stand still and look directly ahead.

Read the weight, record on client's card and inform the client.

Body measurement

Measurements to be recorded:

- bust/chest
- waist
- hips
- upper thigh

- lower thigh
- calf
- upper arms

Select a tape measure that is in good condition not frayed or stretched. Always ensure that the tape is level on the part and not twisted. Do not pull the tape measure. Use the nearest prominent bony point as a marker; this will ensure that the tape will be placed at the same level each time. Thin elastic can be used to indicate the level.

Instruct the client to:

- remove clothing and wear pants only; very self-conscious women may keep a bra on but they should wear the same bra each time the measurements are taken
- stand in bare feet
- maintain good posture with the arms to the side.

CHEST

- Bring the tape around the back, under the arm pit and around the nipple line.
- Record measurement and inform client.

WAIST

- Give a circle of narrow elastic to the client and ask her to place this at the narrowest part; ie, her natural waistline.
- Measure just above the elastic.
- For males, measure at the level of the naval.
- Record measurement and inform client.

HIPS

- Place the tape around the widest part of the hips and measure.
- Measure the distance of the tape from the greater trochanter; this will ensure that the tape is placed at the same level next time.
- Record measurement and inform client.

RIGHT AND LEFT UPPER THIGH

- Use a circle of narrow elastic. Place this around the widest part of the thigh.
- Measure the distance from the top of the patella; eg, 8–10 inches.
- Place the tape around leg just above the elastic.
- Record measurement and inform the client.

RIGHT AND LEFT LOWER THIGH

- Use a circle of narrow elastic and place 2–3 inches above the top of the patella.
- Place the tape around the leg just above the elastic.
- Record measurement and inform the client.

RIGHT AND LEFT UPPER ARMS

- Place a circle of narrow elastic around the widest part of the upper arm.
- Measure the distance from this to the olecranon process.
- Place the tape around the arm, just above the elastic.
- Record measurement and inform client.

MIDRIFF

- For clients whose objective is to lose body weight, measurement of the midriff is necessary.
- Measure 2–3 inches below the xiphoid process.
- Record measurement and inform the client.

CALF

- For those wishing to build up the calf muscle, measure around the widest part of the calf and note the distance from tape to the lateral malleolus. Use this distance next time.
- Record measurement and inform the client.

Testing for muscle strength

Muscle strength is measured by how much weight the muscle is able to move. This is tested using weights, a grip test or pulling against machines.

Weight lift

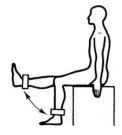

Figure 14.2 *Quadriceps strengthening test*

- Select a suitable stable starting position.
- Select an appropriate weight and check that it is secure.
- Isolate the movement to the muscle being tested.
- Lift the weight smoothly to full inner range, three times. If an extra lift is possible, the weight must be increased.
- Rest for one to two minutes and repeat with extra weight.
- The weight that is lifted smoothly two to three times indicates the strength of the muscle.
- Record the weight.

Power lifters will test the weight that can be lifted once.

Grip test

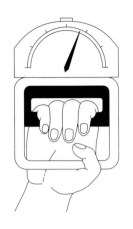

- Hold a grip dynamometer comfortably in the hand.
- In the standing position, lift the arm above the head.
- Lower arm and squeeze as hard as possible.
- Repeat three times.
- Record the highest reading.

Figure 14.3   *Grip test*

Weight machines

There are a variety of machines on the market designed for testing muscle strength. Read the manufacturer's instructions very carefully; test on yourself or a colleague to ensure that you fully understand the procedure.

Exercises such as push ups and sit ups are sometimes used to give an indication of fitness, but these are not measurable.

Muscle tone

It is possible to obtain some indication of muscle strength by applying manual resistance to muscle action and feeling the degree of *tone* within the muscle. This will only provide a rough guide as it is not possible to quantify the strength. It is only possible to categorise it into poor, good, very good or excellent. Muscles easily tested in this way are biceps and triceps, the abdominals, gluteus maximus, the hip abductors and adductors, and the quadriceps.

- Position the client in crook lying. This position can be maintained throughout and avoids moving the client unnecessarily.
- One hand must be placed over the working muscle to feel the increasing tone, the other hand is used to resist the movement.

BICEPS

- The client bends the elbow to mid point of range.
- Place one hand over biceps on the anterior aspect of the upper arm.
- Grasp the wrist with the other hand.
- Instruct the client to bend the elbow while you stop the movement.
- Feel the increased tone with the hand placed over the muscle. Is the power you are feeling poor, good, very good, excellent? This value judgement becomes easier with practice.
- Record the result.

TRICEPS

- Move the hand to cover triceps on the posterior aspect of the upper arm.
- Keep the other hand around the wrist.
- Instruct the client to straighten the elbow.
- Feel the increased tone with the hand placed over the muscle, and judge the power.
- Record the result.

ABDOMINAL (PARTICULARLY RECTUS ABDOMINUS)

- Place one hand over the abdominals.
- Instruct the client to perform a curl up (chin on chest and lift head and shoulders).
- If this is done with ease, the free hand can be placed over the sternum and resistance given to the curl up.
- Feel the increased tone with the hand placed on the abdominals and judge the power.
- Record the result.

GLUTEUS MAXIMUS

- Instruct the client to lift her bottom up off the bed and tighten the buttocks.
- Place a hand over gluteus maximus.
- Feel the increased tone and judge the power.
- Record the result.
- (A sand bag weight can be placed over the pelvis to add resistance.)

ABDUCTORS

- Straighten the client's leg.
- Place one hand over the abductors on the outer aspect of the hip above the greater trochanter.
- Place the other hand under the ankle to cup it.

- Instruct the client to 'push out' towards you.
- Resist the movement using the hand at the ankle pushing inwards.
- Feel the increased tone in the abductors and judge the power.
- Record the result.

ADDUCTORS

- Keep the client's leg straight and pulled outwards.
- Keep the hand under the ankle.
- Place the other hand over the adductors on the inner aspect of the thigh on the upper third.
- Instruct the client to pull the leg inwards towards the other.
- Resist the movement using the hand at the ankle pulling outwards.
- Feel the increased tone in the adductors and judge the power.
- Record the result.

QUADRICEPS

- Straighten the client's leg.
- Place one hand on front of leg above the ankle.
- Place the other hand over the bulk of the quadriceps muscle.
- Instruct the client to tighten the knee and move the patella upwards.
- Feel the tone in the quadriceps with the hand and judge the power.
- Instruct the client to keep the knee straight and lift the leg. Give resistance over the lower leg.
- If a straight leg lift is not possible and the knee gives, the quadriceps muscle is weak.

Cardio-respiratory endurance

This may be tested using a treadmill or bicycle ergo-meter. If this specialised equipment is not available, the step test can be used.

3-minute step test

EQUIPMENT

- 12 inch step
- metronome

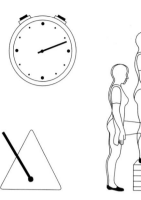

Figure 14.4   *Step test*

■ timing clock/stop watch
■ stethoscope for measuring heart rate or take the pulse.

METHOD

1 Explain the test to the client, demonstrate how to step up and down for 3 minutes at 24 steps per minute.
2 Ask him/her to practise.
3 Set the metronome to 96 clicks per minute for males, 88 clicks per minute for females (with each click a foot must move).
   ■ Click 1: right foot onto step
   ■ Click 2: left foot onto step
   ■ Click 3: right foot down off step
   ■ Click 4: left foot down off step
   Repeat for the 96 clicks of the metronome.
4 Sit and quickly take the client's pulse or heart rate for 1 minute (count for 30 seconds and multiply by 2). The pulse rate is an excellent indication of cardiovascular efficiency. If the recorded heart rate is above the maximal heart rate recommended for that client, the client is unfit and must exercise with caution. As fitness increases and cardiovascular efficiency increases, the heart rate will decrease. As a rough guide, compare the test result with Table 14.1.

Table 14.1   Step test result guidelines

	Men 20–46	**Women 20–46**
Excellent	81–90	79–84
Good	99–102	90–97
Above average	103–112	106–109
Average	120–121	118–119
Below average	123–125	122–124
Fair	127–130	129–134
Poor	136–138	137–145

(Adapted from YMCA 'Ys Way to Fitness'.)

MAXIMUM HEART RATE

To calculate Maximum Heart Rate subtract the age of client from 220 (see page 121). For other specialist equipment, follow the manufacturer's instructions carefully.

Body composition

EQUIPMENT
Skin fold callipers

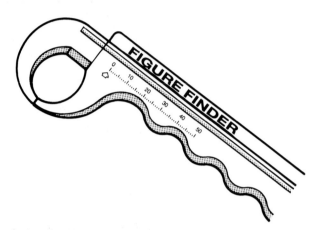

Figure 14.5 *Skin fold callipers*

METHOD

1 Identify the locations for the skin folds; see Table 14.2.
2 Hold the callipers in the dominant hand.
3 Pinch the skin fold with the thumbs and forefinger of the other hand.
4 Hold the calliper perpendicular to the skin fold and place the pads very near the thumb and forefinger.
5 Close or release the callipers depending on type.
6 Record the measurement.
7 Take three or more readings at each skin fold to gain consistency.

Table 14.2 Locations for the skin folds

For women:	For men:
Supra iliac fold diagonally above the crest of the ilium.	Abdominal fold vertically 2 cm lateral to umbilicus.
Anterior thigh fold vertically midway between knee and hip.	Anterior thigh fold vertically midway between hip and knee.
Triceps fold vertically midway between elbow and shoulder.	Chest diagonally half way between nipple and crease of axilla.

The common readings at each site are then averaged and compared with Table 14.3 for recommended body fat.

Table 14.3 Summary of readings

For Women	For Men	Rating
Less than 25 mm	Less than 22 mm	excellent
42 mm–25 mm	34 mm–22 mm	good
65 mm–43 mm	73 mm–35 mm	average
82 mm–66 mm	90 mm–74 mm	fair
Over 82 mm	Over 90 mm	poor

Lung capacity measurement

EQUIPMENT

Spirometer

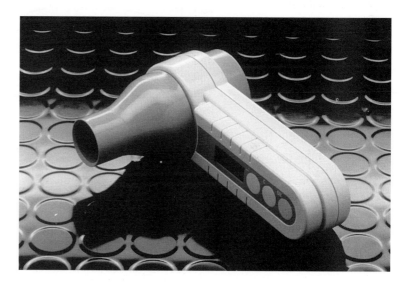

Figure 14.6   *A spirometer*

METHOD

1 Stand straight.
2 Clip on nose clip.
3 Completely fill the lungs with air with deep inhalation.
4 Place mouth around disinfected mouth piece and ensure a perfect seal.
5 Breathe out as hard as possible for as long as possible.
6 Take three attempts to ensure accurate reading, pause for three to four minutes between each attempt.
7 Read and record the measurements and compare with charts for normal ranges.

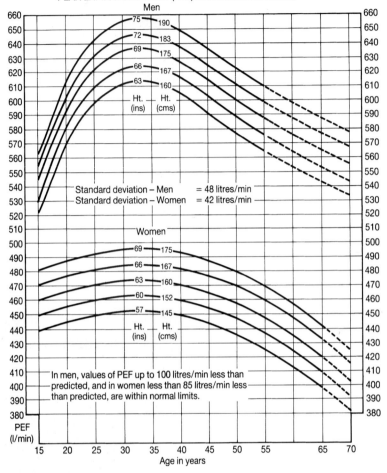

Figure 14.7 *Lung capacity test*

Blood pressure

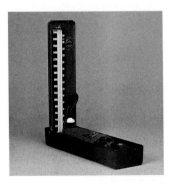

Figure 14.8 *A sphyngmamometer*

EQUIPMENT

This is measured using a *sphygmomanometer*. The modern models usually found in fitness centres are automatic and give a digital readout. These differ from models used medically, where a stethoscope is used over the radial artery at the elbow and the sounds during systole and diastole are listened to and the corresponding pressure level for each is read.

METHOD

1 With automatic models follow the manufacturer's instructions.

2 Normal average blood pressure is:

$$\frac{\text{systolic}}{\text{diastolic}} - \frac{120}{80} \text{ mmHg}$$

3 Abnormally high or low blood pressure should be medically referred.

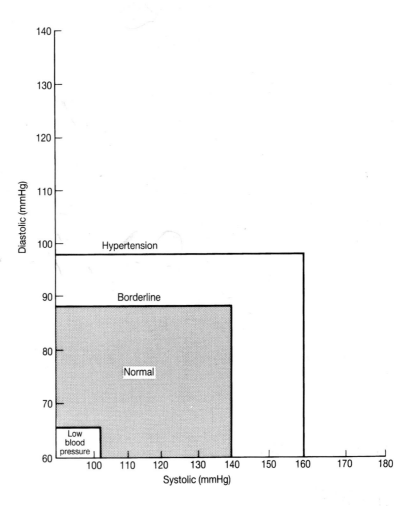

Figure 14.9 *Blood pressure range*

Flexibility

Lower back and hamstring flexibility for the fit client.

EQUIPMENT

A box or stool with a tape attached.

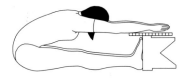

Figure 14.10   *Flexibility test*

METHOD

1 Long sitting with feet against the box or stool.
2 Arms stretched forward.
3 Breathe out, reach and slide the hands along the stool, read the distance at the middle finger.
4 If the box has a slider, push this forward with the hands and take this reading.
5 Take three attempts and record the best result.

Questions

1 List six reasons why accurate assessment is important prior to fitness training.
2 Describe how you would prepare a client for assessment.
3 List the areas which you would measure and record for a client wishing to lose general body fat.
4 Explain how you would test for the strength of the quadriceps muscle using free weights.
5 Explain how you would test the flexibility of the lower back.
6 Explain the procedure when using skin fold callipers for assessing body composition.

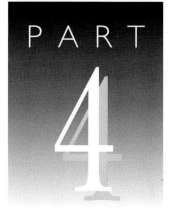

PART

4

Treatments

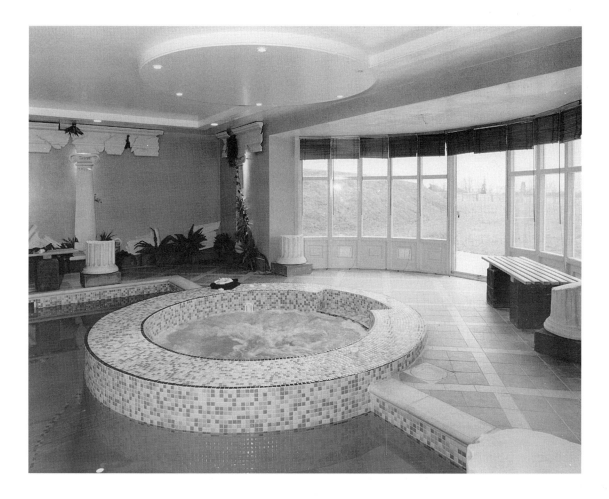

CHAPTER 15

First Aid Treatment

Attempting to diagnose or treat any injury without specialist medical training is dangerous practice. The rate and success of recovery will depend on accurate diagnosis, followed by careful rehabilitation. Inappropriate treatment can cause further damage and permanently impair function. However, knowing what action to take immediately before medical attention is available can reduce the extent of tissue damage. The trainer is often the first person on the scene following injury and must make rapid and crucial decisions based on knowledge and experience. Everyone connected with sport should be familiar with the principles of first aid, as immediate action may be needed.

Prevention of injury

Every precaution should be taken to prevent the occurrence of injury. Factors which contribute to injuries are:

- Inadequate or inappropriate training: plan well designed exercise schemes showing gradual progression, give accurate instruction.
- Inadequate warm up and cool down.
- Faulty equipment and poor surfaces: select a suitable venue with appropriate facilities and good surfaces, check equipment.
- Improper use of equipment.
- Inappropriate footwear or clothing.
- Unsuitable weather conditions.
- Incomplete recovery following a previous injury: ensure adequate rest, relaxation and recovery time.
- Activities inappropriate to age and fitness levels: ensure appropriate fitness assessment prior to undertaking sport or exercise and also on return after injury.
- Intensive competition, resulting in risk taking.

- Dehydration and poor nutrition.
- Exercising when there are contra-indications.
- Poor exercise technique: maintain good body alignment throughout, practise correct technique and breathing patterns.

Immediate assessment of injury

It is vitally important to assess the situation as soon as injury occurs. The injured person should not be moved until a preliminary examination has been carried out.

Breathing

Watch for chest movement or check nose and mouth for air flow. If there is no rise and fall of the chest, and you feel no movement of air, begin mouth to mouth resuscitation.

Heartbeat

Feel for pulse: radial pulse at wrist, carotid pulse at throat behind wind pipe. If there is no pulse, begin cardiac compression.

Broken bones

If for any reason fractures are suspected, do not move the casualty more than is absolutely necessary. This is particularly important if there is damage to the spine. Moving a casualty with damage to their spine can result in permanent paralysis.

Bleeding

Any profuse bleeding should be stemmed by applying firm even pressure directly over the area, preferably over a sterile dressing. Protect yourself from blood contamination.

Other injuries

Look for wounds, cuts abrasions, signs of joint damage; eg, pain, ligament sprains, muscle and tendon strain and tears.

Immediate treatment

The quicker the treatment is administered following injury the greater the chance of speedy full recovery. Treatment should start immediately where possible and certainly within 24 hours.

Treatment is generally aimed to:

- preserve life
- promote healing
- return body to normal function.

More specific aims are:

- to prevent further damage
- to reduce the inflammatory response
- to reduce pain, swelling and stiffness
- to gradually stretch, mobilise and strengthen the affected tissues
- to maintain full strength and condition of unaffected body parts.

Fast action limits damage: for immediate action, think 'RICED':

- **R** – rest and immobilisation to prevent further damage.
- **I** – apply ice immediately for vasoconstriction and to prevent secondary damage.
- **C** – compression to the area to reduce swelling.
- **E** – elevation (using gravity to assist drainage from the area).
- **D** – diagnosis by a doctor either on site, in a surgery or in hospital.

Rest

Further damage to an injured part can be prevented by resting and immobilising the part. The casualty should only be moved if absolutely necessary, to facilitate breathing, to remove from the field of play or to prevent further injury.

The injured part should be rested and supported correctly using splints, tubular, stocking or crepe bandages as necessary. These give firmer support if a layer of cotton wool is wrapped around the area before applying the bandage. If leg fractures are suspected, the good leg can be used as a splint by tying the two legs together, or long strips of wood can be used and bound to the leg until medical treatment is available. A stretcher will then be needed to transport the casualty.

The casualty should rest for 24–48 hours after injury and should not put weight on an injured leg. Elbow or axillary crutches should be used, or support can be given by a person on either side with the casualty hopping on the good leg.

If the arm is seriously injured, a sling should be used for support. A triangular sling is placed around the lower arm and supporting the elbow. The long end is taken over the opposite shoulder and the short end over the injured side, the two ends are tied at the back of the neck. If the injury is below the elbow, the forearm should be supported upwards to assist drainage.

Crutch walking

Measure the crutches carefully. There should be a space the width of 3 fingers (ie, 6 cms) between the top of the crutch and the axilla (arm pit), otherwise pressure will damage the nerves in the region. The hand rest should be level with the crease of the wrist or the styloid process.

Two point walking should be used when both crutches are moved forward together: the casualty pushes on the hand rest, straighten the elbows and hops to the crutches – do not hop *through* the crutches as this can result in loss of balance and falling backwards. Do not place the crutches too far forward as they will slip. The rhythm will be

- lift and move crutches forward
- push on hands
- straighten elbows
- hop to the crutches.

For going upstairs, put foot first, then crutches; for coming downstairs, put crutches first, then foot.

Elbow crutches are used in a similar way, but do not give as much support.

Ice

(See Chapter 16 for technique.)

Ice should be placed over the injured area as soon as possible. This will reduce the metabolic rate and oxygen requirement of the cells around the periphery of the injury. These cells would not receive oxygen because of the damage to blood vessels and would die resulting in secondary injury. Cold will also reduce internal bleeding and swelling as the blood vessels constrict, reducing fluid exudate and bruising.

Care must be taken when applying ice to the area, as there is a risk of producing ice burns if the ice comes into contact with the skin over a prolonged period. The area should be covered with oil for ice cube massage, or a tea towel should be used between the skin and the ice when using ice packs.

There are various ways of applying ice:

1 Stroke the oiled skin with an ice cube, keeping the ice moving over the area slowly.
2 Ice cubes can be shattered and placed in a towel, which is wrapped around the injury over a tea towel.
3 Freezer packs or even frozen food such as a packet of peas can be used; place them over a tea towel covering the area, and hold in place by another towel. These packs are very useful as they can be refrozen and reused.
4 Ankle and wrist injuries can be immersed in iced water in a bucket or bowl. The part is held in the water for as long as is tolerable, is removed for a few minutes and then re-immersed.

Ice should be applied for at least 10–15 minutes, increasing to 30 minutes, unless the skin is sensitive and the area feels uncomfortable. The skin should turn colour: pink for pale skin but darker for dark skin.

Ice should be applied every two to three hours, initially working down to three times a day as healing progresses and the swelling subsides.

Note: Heat should never be used in the acute stage of injury as it increases metabolic rate, and produces vasodilation, which increases blood flow and swelling. Heat may be used after healing has taken place (usually in 6–12 days), but only after the bruising turns yellow.

Compression

This means applying pressure to the area, which helps to limit the bleeding into the tissues. An elasticated tubular or crepe bandage may be used. Additional pressure can be applied if a layer of cotton wool is applied to the area before bandaging. Do not use non-elasticated bandages on a recent injury; the strapping needs some stretch to allow for swelling.

The strapping must not be too tight, as it will restrict the circulation. If the swelling increases, the pressure under the strapping will increase, and this will produce further restriction and damage. Check the swelling and the colour of the skin and nails beyond the strapping; white/grey skin and blue nails indicate that the strapping is too tight, in which case the bandage should be released.

Elevation

The injured part should be supported in elevation whenever possible. Gravity will then assist the drainage of any fluid exudate away from the area. This will help to reduce the pressure within the tissues and the pain around the damaged area.

Diagnosis

Accurate diagnosis is crucial for maximum recovery. Seek medical advice as quickly as possible if there is doubt about the injury, and for any of the following conditions:

- Head injuries
- Headache, nausea, vomiting, dizziness following head injuries
- Pains in the neck or symptoms down the arms such as tingling or numbness
- Pains in the back and down the legs, or numbness
- Breathing difficulties or pains in the chest
- Fracture or suspected fracture
- Dislocation of a joint, or severe injury to a joint or ligament
- Profuse bleeding and deep or large wounds
- Severe muscle and tendon injuries

- Abdominal or groin pain
- Eye injuries.

Summary of precautions

- Do not move a casualty with injuries to the spine.
- Do not move a casualty with fractured bones, more than is absolutely necessary.
- Apply bandages and strapping firmly, but not too tightly as too much pressure may restrict the circulation.
- Check the limbs beyond the strapping for cold, white or blue colouration which indicates lack of circulation – loosen the strap immediately if this is the case.
- Do not apply heat in any form to the injured area; ie, do not use heat lamps, hot packs, hot baths, showers, ultra sound, diathermy, hot towels or any liniments.
- Do not massage the injured area.
- Do not exercise through the pain or use electrical stimulation.
- Do not allow the injured person to drink alcohol.

Types of injury

Injuries can be divided into two categories:

1 *Acute injuries:* Traumatic injuries which happen suddenly due to some external force or internal stress; these produce sudden pain, swelling, bruising or wounds.
2 *Chronic injuries:* Repetitive strain injuries or overuse injuries occur slowly and become progressively worse over a period of time. Pain and swelling is usually of gradual onset but persists over a long period of time.

Skin and subcutaneous tissues injuries

Sharp objects, equipment or apparatus, the playing surface etc. may cause injuries to the skin and underlying tissue. These include cuts, abrasions, infections, contusions, blisters.

When dealing with blood spill injuries, protect yourself from contact with blood. Wear rubber surgical gloves if available, or place the contact hand in a plastic bag. This is important procedure as many life threatening viruses are transmitted through blood contamination.

Cuts

Cuts should be thoroughly cleaned and all dirt or debris removed. They should be washed or swabbed with clean water and/or antiseptic solutions, then covered with a sterile dressing. Swab from the centre outwards and use a clean area each time the wound is touched. Cover with a sterile dressing and bandage in position.

Small cuts can be covered with plasters but again clean carefully, dry and apply the gauze centre over the cut. For stab type cuts, draw the edges together with butterfly plasters. If there is extensive bleeding from a wound, cover with a sterile dressing and apply pressure with a cotton wool pad; bandage and elevate the area. Seek medical treatment as soon as possible. Large cuts over 2 cm long and gaping will require stitching – refer at once to a Casualty Department.

Abrasions

These are caused by friction or scraping of the skin, and are usually superficial. Clean and treat as cuts.

Infections

Cuts and abrasions can become infected as a result of dirt and micro-organisms penetrating the skin or hair follicles. Infections may result in boils or carbuncles which may require antibiotics to prevent them spreading to underlying tissues. Refer to a doctor if infection occurs.

Contusions

Contusion is caused by a direct blow, and results in bleeding into the tissues. Apply ice directly over the contusion to reduce bleeding and swelling. Do not use heat or massage, as these will increase bleeding.

Blisters

Blisters are the result of pressure or friction, and prevention is better than cure. If blisters have developed, they should be left intact as the skin acts as a barrier to infection. A blister can be protected from pressure by surrounding it with a piece of plastic foam with a hole in the middle, then protected with adhesive plaster and left to heal. Large blisters or blood blisters which cause pain due to the build up of pressure can be carefully punctured. Use a sterile needle and puncture two tiny holes in the blister. Gently squeeze out the fluid and cover with a non-adhesive sterile dressing and then plaster.

If the area is raw, clean it with water and apply an antiseptic gel or plastic skin. Use sterile equipment to avoid infection.

Muscle injuries

Injuries to muscles may be strains, partial tears or complete tears, and haematoma.

Strains

Strains will damage and result in micro tears within some fibres of the muscle. The symptoms of pain and stiffness are slow in onset and usually mild. Active movement or passive stretching will cause pain around the damaged area.

Partial tears

These result in tearing and disruption of some fibres within the muscle. The symptoms are felt immediately with severe pain and tenderness, especially when attempting to contract the muscle.

Complete tears

These involve the tearing of all muscle fibres, and the two ends of the muscle contract away from each other. Pain, swelling and tenderness is very severe and there will be complete loss of function. This type of injury may require surgery – refer quickly to hospital.

Muscular haematoma

Direct impact injuries will result in muscle rupture and bleeding. Bleeding may occur within a muscle (intramuscular) or between muscles (intermuscular). It is important to diagnose these injuries accurately as recovery from intermuscular haematoma should be relatively quick and complete. However, complications can arise following intramuscular haematoma due to intracompartmental pressure; muscle function may be absent and recovery may be slow and incomplete.

Initially, muscle injuries should be treated with RICE as soon as possible and continued for 48–72 hours. Any vigorous movements, stretching, heat and massage must be avoided initially, as complications may result.

Tendon injuries

Tendons attach muscles to bone. Tendon injuries are either ruptures (tears) or inflammation (tendinitis).

Tears

Tendons usually tear at their weakest point, ie, where they join the muscle at the musculo-tendinous junction. They may be *partial* tears, when some fibres are torn or *complete* tears when the tendon is severed. Pain may be mild or severe.

Complete tears may require surgery and the best results are obtained if surgery is performed immediately, before the two ends shrink and move apart. Pain is immediate, sharp and severe. It feels like a sharp blow or a 'snap' sensation in the area; the 'snap' can sometimes be heard.

Tendinitis

Inflammation of a tendon (tendinitis) and inflammation of the tendon in its sheath (tenosynovitis) are very common problems. They are usually caused by repetitive stress or overuse, but can be caused by awkward movements such as landing awkwardly or mis-hitting a ball. The pain is niggling and comes on gradually. It is worse when the tendon is moved and may progress until movements are impossible. Because the blood supply to tendons is poor, they can take a very long time to heal: up to 12 weeks or even longer.

Ligaments

Ligaments attach bone to bone; they support and stabilise joints. Ligaments are damaged when joints are forced into abnormal positions. Ligaments may be sprained, partially or completely torn.

Sprained

This occurs when a few fibres are torn, producing pain and swelling. These heal quickly with little disruption of joint movement.

Partial tears

Many fibres are torn because of greater stress. These produce severe pain and swelling, and the joint will be unstable.

Complete tears

These are very severe, producing extreme pain and swelling; the joint will be quite unstable and may dislocate. Torn ligaments may heal well without surgery but others require suturing (a stitch or stitches for closing a wound, or joining two or more structures).

Injuries to ligaments result in bruising, tenderness and swelling around the affected joint, and the healing process may take over six weeks. The joint should be supported during this time with some form of strapping. Severe tears may require a brace or plaster cast.

Menisci

These are discs of cartilage found in certain joints such as the knee, where the medial and lateral menisci lie on the upper surface of the condyles of the tibia. These may tear due to excessive forces during rotation or extreme flexion, causing acute pain and swelling. The knee may lock if a part of the discs becomes dislodged as it may interfere with the function of the knee. Surgery may be required to remove part of the cartilage but some tears heal without surgery.

Bursae

These are sacs of fluid which reduce friction between moving parts of a joint. They may lie between tendons and bones to allow smooth movement of the tendon over the bone. They usually become inflamed because of overuse or repetitive trauma.

Inflammation of a bursa is known as *bursitis*: it produces pain and swelling in the area of the bursa and radiates pain around it. It may heal with rest or may require a cortisone injection to help it settle. Very occasionally surgery is required for a chronic, persistently painful bursa.

Bone fractures

A fracture is a break in a bone. It may be classified as transverse, oblique, spiral or comminuted. Fractures may be *simple* or *compound*:

- A simple fracture is a clean break in the bone with the skin intact.
- A compound fracture involves more complex breaks of the bone and perforation of the skin.

Bones fracture due to excessive force applied to the bone. Stress or fatigue fractures occur as a result of overuse, when repetitive muscle contraction pulls on the bone. This causes repeated minor stress and damage which does not have time to heal. Fractures require immobilisation to reduce the displacement and prevent movement, thus allowing time for the fracture to heal. Fractures of the upper limb usually heal in six to eight weeks, providing there are no complications such as inadequate blood supply. However, limb fractures take 12 to 14 weeks. Fractures heal more quickly in children than adults.

Treatment of soft tissue injuries

These are general guidelines; treatment will vary depending on the type and extent of the injury. Only those with specialist knowledge should attempt to treat sports injuries.

1 *Acute phase:* for immediate treatment, apply RICED; ice applications should be used every hour and then every two to three hours.

Slow static movements within the limit of the pain can be practised two to three times a day. These isometric movements must be performed slowly, and must stop before pain is felt. Start with three contractions only, then build up gradually to five, seven and ten, providing there is no deterioration in the condition.

2 *Sub-acute phase* (24–48 hours): continue with the above routine. Once static movements can be carried out without pain, add gentle active movements within the painfree range. When inner and middle range is painfree, move into outer range; it is important to maintain flexibility.

No definite timescale can be set for these stages, they will depend on the extent of the injury and the speed of recovery.

Rehabilitation

Stage 1

This will begin as soon as possible after severe pain and muscle spasm eases. It is a non-weight bearing phase; ice or other modalities may be used. Free active exercises must be practised four to six times per day. Little and often is the best format – the number must increase each time. Eccentric work may be easier initially. Static stretch exercises should also be included to improve flexibility. During this phase, the unaffected parts should be exercised to maintain fitness levels, but care must be taken not to stress the injury.

Stage 2

This is a partial weight bearing phase, which will begin when there is little swelling and no pain in nearly full range of movement. Heat can now be used, or other modalities. Muscles are exercised against light resistance with a build up of repetitions. Partial weight bearing exercises are practised; pain must be the guide – if it hurts, stop.

Stage 3

This is the weight bearing phase. Strength training, flexibility and co-ordination work are included, in preparation for the return to normal activities.

Stage 4

This is a return to full function. This phase must be planned to cover all the activities that the client will encounter on return to normal situation, whether simply coping with daily living or heavy training. Much encouragement is required in this stage as movements which caused the injuries must be introduced.

It is important not to progress too quickly through each phase as injuries may recur if athletes are over anxious to return to their sport. Fitness tests must be undertaken to ensure adequate fitness levels before resuming sporting or normal activities.

Common injuries

While it is not possible to cover all injuries and their treatment in this book, examples of common injuries are included. Students who require more detailed knowledge must refer to specific medical books.

Foot and ankle joint

Injury	Description	Treatment
Stress fractures	Caused by repetitive stress to the small bones of the foot due to long distance running, marching etc. Pain over the site of the fracture	RICED. Stop activity until healing is complete. Wear shoes with adequate firm sole.
Plantar fasciitis	The fascia on the sole of the foot becomes inflamed. Caused by change of footwear, excessive or different movements performed by the foot. Pain just in front of, or over the heel.	RICED. A sponge shock absorber under the heel may help.
Spring ligament strain	Caused by over stretching of the spring ligament in the sole of the foot, through excessive walking, running, jumping etc. Pain is felt in the sole.	RICED. Wear well supporting shoes; arch support may help.

Injury	Description	Treatment
Bursitis	Inflammation of the bursa between the Achilles tendon and calcaneus, caused by rubbing of ill fitting shoes. Pain and tenderness felt at the back of the heel.	RICED. Change footwear, making sure heel tab is low and not rubbing.
Achilles tendon, partial or complete rupture	Partial tearing of the tendon caused by sudden stretching when muscles are cold or tired. Sudden pain felt over the tendon or in the calf. Complete rupture of the tendon again caused by severe stretching of the tendon when muscles are tired or cold. A sudden severe pain is felt in the calf, as though you have just been kicked. Walking is very difficult, standing tip toe on one leg is impossible.	RICED. May take six weeks to heal; use massage and gentle stretch to recover normal function. RICED. Seek medical advice immediately as surgery is nearly always necessary to suture the ends of tendon together.
Tendinitis and tenosynovitis	Inflammation of the tendons, or tendons and their sheaths. Pain and tenderness felt along the tendon. Stiffness develops and 'crepitus' (a grating sound) may be heard as the tendon moves in the sheath. Caused by excessive use of the tendon or rubbing of ill fitting shoes. May occur to any of the tendons around the foot or wrist.	RICED. May take six weeks or more to settle. Avoid all activities that produce pain and crepitus.
Tendon strain	May occur to any of the long tendons around the foot and ankle. Pain is felt along the tendon.	RICED. Wear well fitting shoes with good support. Ensure good technique and adequate warm up.
Sprained ankle	A very common injury which may affect the medial ligament of the ankle but more usually affects the outer lateral ligament, as there is a greater range of movement when turning foot inwards (inversion). It occurs when the foot 'turns over'. Pain and tenderness is felt over the site of the injury; there may be bruising and swelling depending on the extent of the injury. The ligaments may rupture and the malleoli may fracture.	RICED. It is important to obtain an accurate diagnosis quickly as the ankle may need strapping or a plaster cast. Ice and elevation must start immediately and continue for 48 hours or more. Crutches may be needed to take weight off the ankle.

Injury	Description	Treatment
Unstable ankle	Following ankle sprains, the ankle may 'give way' at times because full function has not returned.	An accurate diagnosis is essential. Strapping may be necessary. Exercises to strengthen the surrounding muscles.
Fractures	Severe trauma can cause a fracture of either fibular or tibial malleolus, or both may fracture. There will be pain, swelling and bruising. All movement of the ankle will hurt and it may be impossible to walk.	RICED. Immediate diagnosis is required; strapping or plaster cast is applied to prevent further damage. Operations are sometimes needed to pin the bones.
Footballer's ankle	Pain and stiffness of the ankle as a result of repeated trauma and kicks to the ankle. The ligaments are damaged and new bone spurs may develop.	RICED. Use of strapping and shin pads to protect against further injury.
Blisters	Caused by rubbing of ill fitting shoes or by excessive activities.	Allow the blister time to heal. Keep the area clean to avoid infection. Check and change shoes if necessary.

Lower leg

Injury	Description	Treatment
Muscle pain and strain	This may happen to any of the muscles of the lower leg. Anterior pain or strain of the muscles in front of the shin, which dorsi flex the foot. Posterior pain or strain of the muscles of the calf which plantar flex the foot. Lateral muscle pain or strain of the lateral muscles which pull the foot outwards (eversion). Medial muscle pain or strain of the muscles which pull the foot inwards (inversion).	RICE. Reduce activities and change training schedules. Analyse and develop correct technique.
Shin splints	Pain over the front and outer side of the shin bone. The nagging ache comes on slowly but may develop into	RICED. Return to training very gradually, ensure adequate warm up and

Injury	Description	Treatment
	a deep pain and extreme tenderness. The constant and repetitive pulling of the muscles on the tibia produces microscopic tearing of the muscle attachments. It is caused by many factors including inadequate warm up, lack of flexibility, poor technique, overuse, fatigue, working or running on hard surfaces.	flexibility, work on spring floors and proper tracks. Wear well supporting, cushion soled shoes.
Stress fractures	Similar to shin splint pain. Caused by repetitive stress to the tibia as above. The bone cracks and is not given the chance to heal.	RICED. Rest for six weeks or more. May need immobilisation in plaster. Return to training very gradually as above.
Simple and compound fractures	The tibia or fibula may fracture, depending on the nature of the injury caused by direct trauma to the lower leg. They are common in soccer and rugby players.	RICED. Seek diagnosis immediately. Will need plaster cast and sometimes surgery. Recovery can take three months or more.
Pain over the tibial tubercle	This is the point of attachment of the quadriceps tendon, therefore pain is caused by excessive sudden pull of the tendon; eg, during deep squats or weight lifting. It may also be caused by long distance running. Pain is felt over the tubercle and also within the muscle when it contracts. The tendon may tear or may pull away a flake of bone.	RICED. Allow sufficient time to heal and avoid stress on the tendon.

Knee injuries

The knee has a complicated hinge structure and is vulnerable to numerous injuries both internal and external. Sudden severe swelling indicates a severe type of injury such as complete rupture of ligaments, or the cartilage or a fracture. Slow swelling over 12 hours or more indicates less severe trauma such as torn cartilage, sprained ligaments or damage of the synovial membrane.

Injury	Description	Treatment
Medial ligament sprains and tears	Pain is felt on the inner side of the knee. It may be mild or severe pain, caused by forcing the lower leg outwards. Fibres may stretch, tear or completely rupture. Frequently happens when skiing and in football, during a tackle or slipping when running. More common than lateral ligament injuries.	RICED. Immediate diagnosis. It may need splinting, plaster cast or surgery depending on severity of the injury.
Lateral ligament sprains and tears	This is the same as the above, except that it occurs when the lower leg is forced inwards and the pain is felt on the lateral aspect of the knee.	RICED. Usually less severe than medial ligament injury.
Dislocation of the patella	The knee cap is forced sideways out of alignment. Caused by a sudden twist on a straight knee or a blow to the knee. Frequently occurs in children. A sharp pain is felt, the knee gives way, this is followed by swelling. May recur, do not force back into place.	RICED. Immediate diagnosis needed as it may require reduction and splinting. Build up the quadriceps muscle to prevent recurrence.
Cartilage injury	This is a very common injury of one or both the menisci, ie, the semilunar cartilage of the knee. It usually occurs by twisting the body on a bent weight-bearing knee or sitting back on the haunches with the feet splayed outwards and rocking backwards. Pain is felt and the knee may give way or lock. Gradual swelling will follow. It may be impossible to straighten the knee.	RICED. Seek immediate diagnosis. The tear may be severe and require keyhole surgery to remove part of the cartilage, or it may heal and recover without surgery. Build up quadriceps before resuming normal activity.
Cartilage ligament injury	The ligament which attaches the cartilage to the edge of the joint may be pinched between the tibia and femur and become inflamed. Caused by incorrect technique when running.	Reduce activity, reassess and modify technique.
Cruciate ligament rupture	The anterior and posterior cruciate ligaments play a vital role in the stability of the knee. They prevent forward and backward movement of the knee. They will tear if the leg is	RICED. Seek immediate medical advice as surgery may be required to suture the ligaments. Strengthen all the muscles around the joint

Injury	Description	Treatment
	severely twisted or forced backwards when weight bearing. One or both cruciates may tear, depending on the force of the injury. Other ligaments may tear at the same time. Severe injury will cause pain swelling and the knee feels floppy.	before resuming activities. After surgery and rehabilitation it is wise to avoid contact sports.
Muscle strains and tears	These can happen to any of the thigh muscles, the quadriceps on the front of the thigh, the hamstrings on the back of the thigh or the adductors on the medial aspect. Muscle *strains* may occur due to over use when muscles become tired and less efficient. Pain develops gradually with tenderness and stiffness but without swelling or bruising. Muscle *tears* may be partial tears or complete ruptures depending on the severity of the blow or injury. Pain is immediate and searing with varying degrees of swelling and bruising.	RICED. Avoid the activity causing the problem and begin rehabilitation. Ensure adequate warm up, stretch and introduce activity gradually. Muscle tears and ruptures must be referred to a doctor as they may require surgery.
Direct blow injuries	These may be caused by a kick or blow from apparatus etc. They vary in severity, depending on the strength of the blow. If the muscle is contracted at the time of the blow, the fibres may tear. Pain is immediate; stiffness and swelling follows. There may be severe internal bleeding, forming a haematoma. If this heals with some bone formation there will be some functional loss.	RICED. Seek immediate diagnosis. The success of the recovery depends on early treatment.
Fractures	Considerable force is required to fracture the large femur but it may occur as a result of violent injury. The surrounding muscles and skin may also be damaged.	Immobilise and seek medical advice immediately.

The pelvis

The pelvis is a very stable structure, formed by the two innominate bones and the sacrum. Problems may be felt around the hip joint, in the groin, over the pubic symphysis or over the coccyx.

Injury	Description	Treatment
Footballer's groin	Inflammation at the symphysis pubis. The ligament may be strained due to movement sideways, ie, side-stepping, hurdling, slipping. Pain is felt over the pubic bone.	Rest, avoid activity which caused the problem.
Adductor strain	Similar to the above and caused in same way but pain is deep in the groin and upon adduction.	RICE. Then gradual stretch of adductors.
Pain in hip joint	May be due to a number of conditions such as osteo-arthritis, bursitis etc.	Refer to doctor for accurate diagnosis.
Coccydynia	Pain at the very base of the spine usually due to a fall on the tail. May be caused by persistent trauma such as practising excessive sit-ups on a hard floor.	Apply ice immediately. May take a long time to heal, seek medical advice if pain persists.

Shoulder and arm injuries

The shoulder joint is a loose fitting ball and socket joint, which allows a wide range of movement. It has a loose capsule and numerous tendons which support the joint.

Injury	Description	Treatment
Muscle strain tears and ruptures	The muscles and tendons around the joint may be strained gradually through overuse or strained suddenly through direct injury. Overuse injuries occur in swimming, rowing, tennis, shot putting, bowling or weight lifting. Traumatic injuries occur in gymnastics, riding, pole vaulting, parachuting etc. The muscles may be strained, partially torn or completely ruptured and the pain and stiffness will vary accordingly.	RICED. Rest from the activity which caused the injury is essential until healing has taken place. A sling may be necessary. Build up strength gradually before resuming activity.

Injury	Description	Treatment
Dislocated shoulder	The capsule of the shoulder is loose and the head of the humerus can be wrenched out of the shallow glenoid cavity. Extreme pain is felt immediately and movement is limited or impossible. Caused by forcing the arm outwards away from the body. Common injury in rugby and judo.	Seek medical advice immediately as the joint needs to be reduced (put back). A sling should be worn for three to six weeks, then build up strength gradually.
Fractures	Any of the shoulder, girdle or arm bones may fracture. Common fractures are those of the clavicle, surgical neck of the humerus, distal end of the radius, scaphoid, ribs. Immediate pain is felt following the trauma, with swelling and bruising, depending on the type of fracture.	Refer immediately to a doctor or hospital Casualty Department.
Frozen shoulder	Inflammation of the lining of the shoulder joint. May be caused by repetitive trauma. Pain and stiffness of the shoulder and movement becomes increasingly limited.	RID. Seek medical advice as other therapies are effective. Can be very slow to recover, from two months to two years.
Bursitis	Inflammation of the various bursae around the shoulder joint, eg, sub deltoid, subacromial or of the olecranon bursa at the elbow. Will produce pain and stiffness around the joint.	RID. Seek medical advice as other therapies are effective. Injection may be needed.
Tennis elbow	Strain of the common extensor tendon over the lateral epicondyle of the humerus. Caused by wrenching, repetitive stress, incorrect technique. Pain is felt over the lateral epicondyle because the tendon becomes inflamed at its attachment. It hurts to extend the wrist with a bent elbow or when straightening the elbow. Affects tennis players, badminton players, and throwers. May occur following any repetitive stress such as lifting, chopping wood or using a screwdriver.	RI. Rest from the activity and ice. It may need an injection of cortizone or operation to release the tendon if the condition persists.

Injury	Description	Treatment
Golfer's elbow	The same as tennis elbow but this is inflammation of the flexor tendon attachment on the medial epicondyle of the humerus. Caused by overuse and stretching of the muscles. Common problem for golfers or javelin throwers. Pain is felt over the medial epicondyle.	RI. Rest from activity and ice. It may need anti-inflammatory injection if condition persists.
Tendinitis and tenosynovitis	Inflammation of the tendons within their sheaths as they pass over the wrist. Pain and tenderness is felt along the tendon and 'crepitus' may be heard. Movement is painful. Caused by over use, repetitive movements and faulty technique.	RID. Rest and ice, avoid unnecessary movements. A splint may be necessary to provide support.
Sprained wrist	Caused by excessive stress and movement of the wrist. The ligaments are sprained with pain and swelling.	RICED. Strapping or splinting may be necessary. May require plaster cast. Resume movement very slowly.

Many other injuries can affect the hand and wrist. Always seek medical advice as function may be impaired through lack of correct treatment.

Chest injuries

Injury to the chest may result in the fracture of one or more ribs. It is unusual to suffer muscle strain unless it accompanies rib fractures.

Range of injuries

- Fractures of ribs.
- Stress fractures of ribs.
- Fractures of the sternum.

Causes

- All fractures are caused by severe stress, such as falling awkwardly and hitting the chest on some hard object, being hit by a cricket or tennis ball.
- Stress fractures are caused by repetitive stress and strong over use of chest muscles as in tennis or shot putting.

Action

- Seek medical advice for accurate diagnosis. Little is done for fractured ribs as they are well held by the intercostal muscles.
- Fractured ribs may sometimes puncture the underlying lung, in which case the casualty should be taken to hospital immediately.

Injuries to the vertebral column

Any area of the vertebral column is susceptible to injury, but most injuries are sustained in the lumbar and cervical regions.

Range of injuries

- Fractures of the vertebrae.
- Strains and tears of the supporting ligaments.
- Strains and tears of supporting muscles.
- Damage or prolapse of the inter vertebral discs.

Causes

- Fractures are usually caused by severe stress such as falling from a height, motor accidents, parachute jumping, hard rugby tackles.
- Tearing of ligaments and muscle fibres is caused by sudden overload.
- Strains and sprains are caused by repetitive stress overload, or by awkward or inappropriate movements.
- Disc damage is caused by sudden increased compression forces; eg, when lifting heavy weights, lifting at an awkward angle, or taking poor postural care during exercise and movement. Trunk forward flexion exercises can damage the lumbar spine and head circling exercise can damage the cervical spine. See Chapter 12.

Action

All severe back injuries must be approached with great care. *Do not move* the casualty unless it is essential to resuscitate and save life. The spinal column protects the spinal cord which runs through the vertebral foramen. Any fracture of the vertebrae can impinge and increase pressure on the cord, can partially damage the cord or can sever it completely. These injuries may result in partial or total paralysis from the level downwards. Moving the casualty will increase the risk of cord damage. Seek medical help immediately. All back injuries must be medically referred. Gradual back pain which becomes progressively worse must also be medically referred.

Questions

1 List six factors which may contribute to injury. Discuss how they may be avoided.
2 Discuss the five checks that you would undertake during the immediate assessment of injury.
3 Explain the RICED principle in the immediate treatment of injuries.
4 Explain why heat should not be given to the area, immediately following injury.
5 List ten conditions which must be medically referred following injury.
6 Define the following:
   A Acute injuries
   B Chronic injuries
7 Explain why rubber gloves should be worn when dealing with any bleeding wounds or pierced skin injuries.
8 Explain how you would treat a blister on the heel.

CHAPTER 16

Cryotherapy

Cryotherapy (cold or ice therapy) is the first line of action in the treatment of sports injury. It is effective, simple, easy to use and inexpensive. It is beneficial in the immediate (acute) post-traumatic phase, and also through the rehabilitation phases. As it is easy to apply with little danger or complication, the athlete can continue the treatment at home. Ice must be applied as soon as possible to the injured part, within 5–15 minutes. Any delay will result in secondary damage which will increase the extent of the injury. This will prolong the rate of recovery and limit the return to full normal function.

Methods of ice application

1 *Ice cubes* which are slowly moved over the area; sometimes referred to as ice massage.
2 *Crushed ice* placed in a plastic or towelling bag; place over the area with a thin towel in between.
3 *Gel freezer packs* which are kept frozen until required and applied to the area as above. These are convenient to use and can be refrozen and reused.
4 *Packs of frozen food* such as peas applied to the area as above; these can be refrozen and reused (but must not be eaten after defrosting).
5 *Chemical packs* which become cold when struck hard to mix the chemicals. These packs are not as effective as other methods as the temperature is not as low. There is also a danger of chemical burns, should the chemicals leak. Manufacturers are continually working on improvements.
6 *Iced water* in a pan or bucket into which the part is immersed. Most suitable for ankle and wrist injuries. To ensure a sufficiently cold temperature, ice must float on the surface throughout the treatment.
7 *Cold aerosol sprays* are not as effective as other methods as they produce superficial cooling only. They do have the advantage of being very convenient, easy to carry around and quick to use.

Physiological effects of cooling the tissues

Certain changes will be produced in the tissues as a result of cold application – these are known as the physiological effects. These effects include:

- a decrease in metabolic rate in the area
- a decrease in the circulation due to vasoconstriction in the area
- local anaesthesia with a reduction in pain
- a decrease in muscle spasm
- a decrease in inflammatory response
- a decrease in the flexibility of ligaments and tendons.

Decrease in metabolic rate

This is the main reason for applying ice to the area immediately following injury. Cold reduces the metabolic rate of cells and consequently their oxygen requirement. If cold therapy is not given, the cells around the periphery of the damaged area will require oxygen to meet metabolic demands. If this demand for oxygen cannot be met because of damage to the blood vessels in the area, the cells will die. This happens within 10–15 minutes following injury and continues for around 12 hours. This will increase the amount of tissue damage and the size of the injury; it is known as 'secondary hypoxic injury'.

By decreasing the cells' metabolic rate and need for oxygen, these cells may survive until circulation is restored, thus limiting the extent of the injury.

Note: The application of heat will have the opposite effect. Heating the tissues will increase metabolic rate and the demand for oxygen, and will cause greater secondary damage. Heat must therefore *not* be used to treat immediate acute injury.

Decrease in circulation

Cold therapy produces vasoconstriction, which will reduce blood flow. Less bleeding into the tissues will facilitate quicker healing. However, the blood clotting mechanism will be activated immediately following injury; this will also prevent blood loss and will have occurred before cold packs can be applied. In addition, the constriction of capillaries in response to cold will reduce fluid exudate and tissue swelling.

Reduction of pain

Cold induces anaesthesia – the sensory receptors in the skin are inhibited and sensation is reduced but not totally absent. Initially (one minute or so after applying the ice) pain is increased. A dull radiating pain is felt which may increase for a while but will eventually pass, giving way to a prickling sensation and then numbness.

The decrease in pain will reduce the attendant muscle spasm and limit the pain–spasm–pain cycle which occurs after injury. This analgesic effect may mask the extent and seriousness of the injury, therefore the athlete or sportsperson must not return to the activity immediately following ice treatment.

Decrease in muscle spasm

It is thought that the reduction in muscle spasm is brought about by the anaesthesia, and because cold decreases nervous transmission and depresses muscle spindle sensitivity and reflex mechanisms. After injury, the body's protective mechanism increases muscle tone to prevent further damage to the tissues. Tight muscles act as a splint preventing movement and hence further damage. If this spasm is inhibited in the early stages, careful active movements can be performed, improving recovery rate. In the rehabilitative stages, less muscle spasm allows greater flexibility and increased range of movement which facilitates a speedier return to full function.

Decreased inflammatory response

It is thought that cold decreases the inflammatory response because it reduces the effects of histamine.

Decrease flexibility of ligaments and tendons

The flexibility of connective tissue decreases after cold application; ligaments and tendons are not as elastic. It is therefore important to stop cold therapy when introducing flexibility exercises. At this stage, when healing is progressing satisfactorily and there is no risk of further bleeding, some form of heat should be given. This may commence 72 hours or so after injury, but the time will depend on the rate of healing and the extent of the injury. If in doubt, continue with ice.

Uses of cryotherapy

1 Cold therapy may be used to treat soft tissue injuries in the acute, subacute, and rehabilitative stages.
2 In the acute stage, ice is applied for 15 minutes every 1–2 hours. Little and often is the best guide. It is most effective at this stage because it slows down the metabolic rate, reduces bleeding and fluid exudate thus limiting further tissue damage.
3 In the sub acute and rehabilitative stages, the time of application is increased to 20–30 minutes, 3–4 times a day. Its main use in these stages is to relieve pain and muscle spasm, and thus facilitate early active movement.
4 To treat overuse injuries.

Contra-indications

- Open bleeding wounds.
- Deficient circulation in the part.
- Lack of skin sensation.
- Hypersensitivity to cold.
- Extreme pain during application.

Factors which affect the rate of cooling

The application of cold to the area conducts heat away from the superficial and deep tissues, resulting in a decrease in temperature. There will be a rapid and immediate reduction in surface temperature, but the temperature of deeper tissues will decrease more slowly and will continue to decrease for some time after the ice is removed. There are many factors which affect the rate of cooling; these include:

1 The area of the part in contact with the ice.
2 The length of time the part is in contact with the ice.
3 The difference in temperature between the part and the ice.
4 The rate at which the body regenerates heat.
5 The rate at which heat is conducted away from the ice.

Ice packs and gel packs used for 30 minutes produce similar cooling effects, but research indicates that immersion in iced water for an equal length of time produces more intense cooling and slower rewarming. This may relate to the larger surface area being treated.

Chemical packs are less effective at reducing temperature than the other methods, and cold sprays produce superficial, temporary cooling only.

Treatment

Remember the RICE routine (rest, ice, compression, elevation).

Ice must be applied as soon as possible, within 5–10 minutes of the injury occurring. Immediate appropriate treatment will increase effectiveness and considerably shorten the recovery period. Ice should be applied as soon as an initial assessment of the injury has been made.

The method of application will depend on availability and convenience. Chipped or crushed ice in a bag, gel packs from a refrigerator, or ice cubes are suitable for most injuries; iced water in a bucket or bowl is suitable for ankle, calf, wrist, forearm and elbow injuries.

If ice is placed in direct contact with the skin it can stick and long-term application can produce ice burns. It is therefore safer to oil the skin lightly before stroking with an ice cube, and to place a thin layer of cold wet towel or bandage on the skin when using an ice pack, ie, between the skin and the ice pack. The part may be immersed in iced water without protection, but if pain is intense the part must be removed from the water for 15–30 seconds and then reimmersed.

Rest is important, as any movement may produce further damage increasing the extent of the injury. Compression may be applied and the part elevated if possible to assist drainage.

Technique using ice pack or gel pack

1 Prepare the ice pack by placing approximately 1 kg of crushed ice in a plastic or towelling bag; alternatively, pile the ice onto the towel and fold the ends over. If using a cold pack, remove from the freezer just before use.

2 Ensure that the client is comfortable, well supported and in a suitable position to receive the treatment.

3 Remove any clothing or jewellery from the area.

4 Explain the treatment to the client, highlighting the beneficial effects and the importance of regular timed application. Explain that pain may be felt or increase initially, but that this will give way to pins and needles and then numbness.

5 Wring out a towel in cold or iced water and place over the injured part. Place the cold pack over this and wrap a double layer of towelling around the part to hold the pack in place. If intense pain develops, the ice must be removed for 15–30 seconds and then reapplied.

6 Compression should be applied and the part elevated and rested.

7 Treat for 15 minutes initially, increasing to 30 minutes in the subacute stage, but this will depend on client tolerance. Pale skin should be red, dark skin will be darker.

8 Repeat the procedure every two hours for the first 24 hours after injury, or as often as possible.

9 Exercise as explained below.

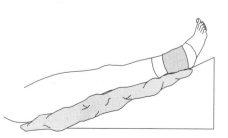

Figure 16.1   *Application of ice packs*

Technique using iced water

1 Fill the container to three quarters full with cold water and ice. Ensure that there is ice floating in the water throughout the treatment.
2 Position the client in a comfortable position; remove all clothing and jewellery around the injury.
3 Explain the treatment to the client as in point 4 above.
4 Immerse the part in the water and reassure that pain is to be expected initially but that it will subside. If the pain is intolerable, lift the part out of the water for 15–30 seconds then reimmerse.
5 Keep the part immersed until it is numb and red; aim for 20 minutes.
6 Remove the part from the water and dry gently.
7 Exercise as explained below.

Technique with ice cube massage

1 Place a supply of ice cubes in a container.
2 Position the client in a comfortable, well supported position; elevate the part if possible.
3 Remove all clothing and jewellery from the area.
4 Explain the procedure to the client.
5 Spread a thin layer of oil over the area.
6 Hold the ice cube with folded tissue or lint.
7 Move the ice slowly over the part, moving up and down in straight lines; overlap the previous stroke. Work over and around the injured part. The ice will melt, so ensure that there is a towel under the part to absorb the water.
8 Continue working in this way for 20 minutes or so, until the part is red and numb.
9 Dry the area gently.
10 Exercise as explained below.

Technique with cold sprays

These aerosol sprays are not as effective as other methods, and are generally used for convenience on the field of play. The part is uncovered and sprayed at a certain distance for a few seconds. It is important that these sprays are used according to manufacturer's directions, as their mode of application may vary. If incorrectly applied they can cause ice burns.

Exercises following cryotherapy

During the first 24–48 hours, ice application is followed by slow, gentle *isometric* exercises. These static muscle contractions are performed within the painfree range.

As healing progresses, *isotonic* movements are performed. The client is instructed to move the joint slowly through to the point just before pain is felt, to hold for a moment and return. All possible joint movements must be practised in this way. Great care must be taken during this subacute stage since movement can disturb the healing process and increase secondary damage.

Remember: movements must not produce pain. All movements must be within the limit of pain.

Example: Treatment to injured ankle joint, where injuries are usually to the lateral or medial ligaments

- Apply cold therapy for up to 30 minutes, then remove.
- Static exercise instruction – 'I'm going to hold your foot firmly and I want you to pull as hard as you can against my hand, stop if there is any pain'. The resistance against the movement must be even, and great enough to produce tension within the muscle but to prevent any movement. Initially the resistance is applied to dorsi flexion (hand applying resistance on the dorsum of the foot), and is then applied to plantar flexion (hand on the sole of the foot). When these contractions are easy to perform, inversion and eversion are added. Exercise away from the injury first; ie, for lateral ligament injury, perform static inversion first. When this is easy, carefully perform static eversion (this may not be possible initially). Each contraction is held for five to six seconds.
  Remember: tension must be developed within the painfree limit.
- After 48–72 hours or so, depending on the severity of the injury, ice treatment is followed by isotonic exercises.
- Instruction for isotonic movement – 'Pull the foot up

slowly towards you (dorsi flexion); stop when you feel any pain; hold; now move the foot slowly down away from you.' (plantar flexion). Repeat for inversion and eversion and then progress to circumduction. Perform three movements of each initially, increasing by two with each application.

Questions

1 List the methods by which ice may be applied.
2 Discuss the physiological effects of cooling the tissues.
3 List the contra-indications to cold therapy.

4 List the factors which affect the rate of cooling.
5 Explain the importance of applying oil to the skin prior to ice massage.
6 State how frequently ice should be administered during the first 24 hours.

Heat Therapy

Many forms of heat therapy are available to the therapist and choice is determined by availability, suitability and client preference. All forms of heat produce similar effects, but some are more suitable for heating small localised areas while others are used for general body heating. The treatment is usually combined with other treatments as part of a routine.

Whether the heat is applied generally or locally, the extent of the effects will be dependent on:

■ the duration of heat application
■ the intensity or degree of the heat
■ the depth of absorption
■ the size of the area being heated.

Methods of heat application

The following methods are used to apply heat to localised areas:

1 Infra red and radiant heat lamps
2 Paraffin wax to specific areas
3 Whirlpool baths
4 Hot packs.

The following methods are used to apply general heat to the body:

1 Sauna
2 Steam baths – individual and communal
3 Spa pools, eg, Jacuzzi
4 Infra red tunnels
5 Various forms of showers.

General contra-indications to heat therapy

1 Areas of defective sensation and hyper sensitive skins
2 Heart conditions and blood pressure disorders

3 Thrombosis or phlebitis
4 Bronchitis, asthma, hay fever or heavy colds and fevers
5 Migraine and headache
6 Skin infections and disorders such as eczema, psoriasis
7 Diabetes
8 Epilepsy
9 After a heavy meal
10 Under influence of alcohol or drugs
11 Later stages of pregnancy
12 First 1–2 days of period especially if heavy
13 Severe exhaustion
14 Recent over exposure to UVL, eg, sunburn

Infra red treatment

Infra red is used by therapists to heat body tissues. It may be used to treat localised areas such as muscle joints, the upper or lower back, or it may be used to heat the body in general.

Infra red rays are electro-magnetic waves, with wave lengths of between 700 nm and 400,000 nm. They are given off from the sun and any hot object, eg, electric fires, gas and coal fires, hot packs and various types of lamps. The lamps that produce infra red rays can be divided into two main types.

1 The non luminous (called **infra red** lamps).
2 The luminous (called **radiant heat** lamps).

Confusion exists regarding these lamps. Both types of lamp emit *infra red rays*. The difference lies in their wave length, which determines their depth of penetration. The non luminous lamp emits rays of longer wave length, around 4,000 nm, while the luminous type emit rays of shorter wave length, around 1,000 nm and include waves from the visible spectrum and UVL. The differing wave lengths produce slightly different effects when absorbed by body tissues.

The non luminous (infra red) lamp

Many types of non luminous lamps are produced; all have a non glowing source that emits infra red rays. A common type uses a coil of wire embedded in fire clay which is placed in the centre of a reflector. When the lamp is

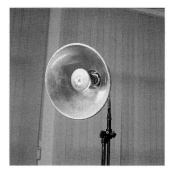

Figure 17.1   *An infra red lamp*

switched on, the wire gets hot and heats the fire clay. The rays are then emitted from the hot fire clay; they pass through the air and are absorbed by a body placed in their path.

The rays from non luminous lamps are of longer wave length, are invisible, less irritating and less penetrating than the short rays from luminous lamps. They may feel hotter at equal distances and power, due to increased absorption in the top layers of the skin.

These wave lengths are further from visible light and are consequently called *far IR*.

The luminous (radiant heat) lamp

These are often called radiant heat lamps, and give off infra red rays from glowing or incandescent sources such as hot wires or powerful bulbs. These are also placed in the centre of a reflector. When the lamp is switched on, the wire glows, giving off infra red and visible rays and small amounts of ultra violet rays. Some bulbs have filters to cut out some visible rays and ultra violet rays – these bulbs are usually red in colour.

The rays produced by these lamps have a shorter wave length, including some visible rays, are more penetrating (down to the subcutaneous layer) and are more irritating than the rays from non luminous lamps.

These wave lengths are nearer visible light and are consequently called *near IR*.

Comparisons of luminous and non luminous lamps

Non Luminous	Luminous
Long wave length around 4,000 nm	Shorter wave length around 1,000 nm
Include no visible rays	Include some visible rays and small amount of UVL
Penetrate approx. 1 mm of skin	Penetrate approx. 3 mm of tissue
Less irritating	More irritating
May feel hotter at equal power and distance	Will feel less hot at equal power and distance
Take 10–15 minutes to heat up	Heat up quickly, approx. 2 minutes

Combined infra red and ultra violet lamps

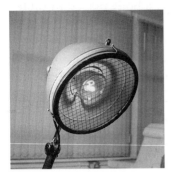

Figure 17.2   *A combined infra red and ultra violet lamp*

Some lamps are manufactured with two elements, one producing UVL rays and the other producing infra red rays. Although these lamps are not generally used by the sports therapist, they are found in some clinics. They can be dangerous in inexperienced or incompetent hands – therapists who do not distinguish between the two may give long duration of UVL, by pressing the wrong switch.

- UVL glows, giving a blue/white colour.
- IR gives invisible rays or glows red/orange.

Ultra violet rays are part of the electro magnetic spectrum, with shorter wave length than infra red rays and visible light rays from 400 nm to 10 nm. These UVL rays are not used for heating effects but for other effects such as tanning.

Manufacturers produce a wide variety of lamps, tunnels and solariums (combined UV), and the therapist should be familiar with all the lamps in the clinic.

- Examine all lamps carefully and read manufacturer's instructions.
- Check stability.
- Check joints and screws for angling the lamp; are they tight and secure?
- How can the angle of the lamp be changed?
- Is there an on/off switch on the lamp or must it be switched on/off at the wall socket?
- Is there an intensity control or must intensity be controlled by increasing or decreasing the distance?
- Is it in good order? Check plugs reflector, grid etc.
- Is it dual purpose, ie, IR and UVL? If so, make sure which switch operates IR and which for UV.

Intensity of radiation

The intensity of radiation will depend on three factors:

1 The intensity of the lamp.
2 The distance between the lamp and the skin.
3 The angle at which the rays strike the part.

The intensity of the lamp

Lamps vary in output and intensity. Some have control dials for increasing and decreasing intensity, others need to be moved further away. The intensity from infra red lamps does not pose any problems, as the client is able to feel if the intensity is too high, and the distance can be increased or lamp turned down.

The distance between the lamp and the skin

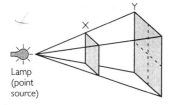

Lamp
(point
source)

Figure 17.3 Radiation from a point source illustrating the law of inverse squares

The Law of Inverse Squares governs intensity in relation to distance. This states that the intensity from a point source (ie, the lamp) varies inversely with the square of the distance from the point source. In other words:

- if the distance increases, the intensity decreases by the square of the distance
- if the distance decreases, the intensity increases by the square of the distance.

Therefore:

- if you double the distance, the intensity is quartered.
- if you reduce the distance by half, the intensity will increase four times (quadrupled).

X is one metre from the source.
Y is two metres from the source.
If the client is placed at distance X, they will receive the calculated dose. If the distance is increased to Y (ie, doubled), the intensity is a quarter of that at X.
To produce the same effect on the skin when changing distances of lamps the following apply.

- If you halve the distance, you quarter the time.
- If you double the distance, you quadruple the time.

The angle at which the rays strike the part

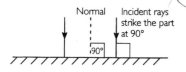

Figure 17.4 The Cosine law

The Cosine Law governs intensity in relation to the angle of incidence. This law states that the intensity of radiation at a surface varies with the cosine of the angle of incidence (ie, the angle between the incident ray and the normal). If the rays strike the part at 90°, the angle of incidence is 0° – there is maximum intensity and penetration. As the incident ray moves down towards the surface, the angle increases and the intensity decreases.

When giving infra red treatments, the lamp should be positioned so that the rays strike the part at 90°. This will ensure maximum intensity, absorption and effect.

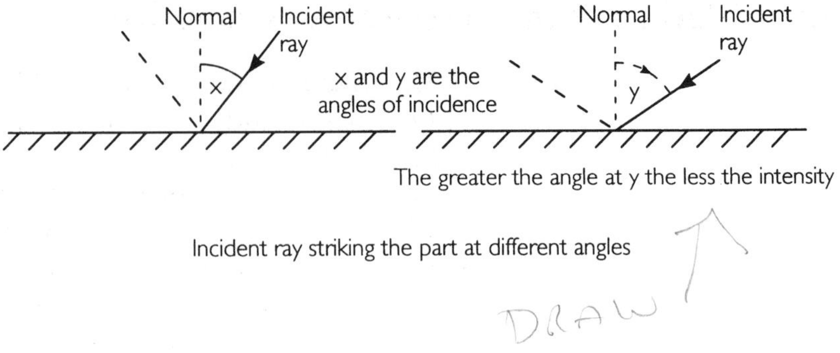

Figure 17.5   *Incident ray striking at different angles*

Incident ray striking the part at different angles

DRAW

Note: Never position lamps directly over the client. The client should be positioned and the lamp angled so that the rays can strike at 90°.

Effects of infra red treatment

Heating of body tissues

When infra red rays are absorbed by the tissues, heat is produced in the area. The rays from luminous generators penetrate more deeply than those from non luminous lamps, therefore superficial and deeper tissues are heated directly. With non luminous lamps, the top 1 mm of skin is heated directly but the deeper tissues are heated by conduction.

Increased metabolic rate

Van't Hoffs Law states that a chemical reaction capable of being accelerated will be accelerated by heat. Metabolism involves many chemical reactions which will be accelerated by heat. The increase in metabolic rate will be greatest where the heating is greatest; with infra red treatment, this will be in the superficial tissues where there will be an increase in cellular activity. More oxygen and nutrients are required and more waste products/metabolites produced. However, if the heating is too prolonged or too intense, protein damage occurs and eventually cell destruction. Therefore gentle mild heating for 15–30 minutes is beneficial but intense heating over 30 minutes can be damaging.

Vasodilation with increase in circulation

- Heat has a direct effect on the blood vessels – it produces vasodilation and an increase in blood flow in an attempt to cool the area.
- Vasodilation is also produced by stimulation of sensory nerve endings, which cause reflex dilation of arterioles.
- Vasodilation is also produced as a result of the increase in metabolic rate and increase in waste products. The metabolites have an effect on the walls of capillaries and arterioles, causing dilation.
- The heat regulating centres of the brain will be stimulated as body heat rises. This will result in general dilation of superficial vessels to ensure that the body is not overheated.
- Increasing the temperature reduces the viscosity of blood, which increases the speed of flow through the vessels.

Hyperaemia is the term used to describe an increase in the flow of blood to the area.
Erythema means reddening of the skin due to vasodilation and hyperaemia.

Fall in blood pressure

General body heating may result in a fall in blood pressure.
If the superficial blood vessels dilate, the peripheral resistance is reduced, and this will result in a fall in blood pressure. (When blood flows through vessels with small lumen, it exerts a certain pressure on the walls. If the lumen is increased by the vessels dilating, the pressure on the walls will be reduced.)

Increase in heart rate

The increased metabolism and circulation means that the heart must beat faster to meet the demand, therefore the heart rate increases.

General rise in body temperature

When one area of the body is heated for a prolonged time, there is a general rise in body temperature by conduction and convection. The heat will be carried to the surrounding tissues by the blood circulating through the area.

Increased activity of sweat glands

As the body temperature rises, the heat regulating centres in the brain are affected. The sweat glands are then stimulated to produce more sweat in order to lose body heat. This increases the elimination of waste products.

Effects on muscle tissue

The skin and subcutaneous fat form a barrier to the conduction of heat, but providing there is little fat, muscle tissue will be warmed by the circulating blood through conduction. The following effects are produced:

1 The rise in temperature reduces muscle spasm, relieves pain and therefore promotes muscle relaxation.
2 The increase in blood flow will provide more nutrients and oxygen which are required for muscle contraction. Warm muscles contract more efficiently than cold muscles. The increase in blood flow will also speed up the removal of the resultant waste products, such as lactic acid.

Effect on joints

Heat may reduce joint pain. This is due to the relaxing effect on the surrounding structures such as muscles and ligaments, to the soothing effect on nerve endings and to the increase in circulation.

Effects on collagenous tissue (ligaments and tendons)

Heat increases the extensibility of collagenous tissue, providing it is simultaneously stretched. Therefore, to improve the range of joint movement, heat and flexibility exercises are effective.

Effects on sensory nerves

Mild heat has a soothing effect on sensory nerve endings. However, intense heat has an irritating effect.

Pigmentation

Repeated and intense exposure to infra red produces a purple or brown mottled appearance on the area. This may be due to destruction of blood cells and release of haemoglobin.

Uses

1 As a general heating treatment to promote relaxation.

2 As a localised treatment for relief of joint pain, muscle spasm, pain and tension.

3 Pre-event to warm the tissues; it must be given for a short time only, around 10 minutes prior to warm up and stretch exercises, but *not* instead of. The aim is to improve flexibility and enhance the contractability of muscles. Too long an application will promote relaxation, which is not required before an event, as the athlete must remain alert and focused. It may be immediately followed by a brisk massage to the appropriate area, and then warm up and stretch exercises must be performed. Used prior to stretch exercises, it increases extensibility of connective tissue components, enhancing flexibility.

4 Post-event to aid the recovery of the tissues; gentle heat used in conjunction with massage will speed up the removal of metabolic waste. This will aid muscle recovery, relieve pain and stiffness, and promote relaxation. It would be given after cool down and stretch exercises. Mild heat only should be used and massage may be performed at the same time. Particular care must be taken when considering the use of heat after an event, because it must not be used if there is any suspicion of inflammation or injury, when ice would be the treatment of choice. Many therapists perform exploratory massage first, in order to assess the condition of the tissues. Ice packs should be used if sore, tender areas are found, but heat would be safe if there were no injuries. Mild heat is given for 15–20 minutes; the massage may continue for 30–40 minutes.

5 After injury to promote healing and recovery; heat should not be given for the first 72 hours after injury as it increases metabolic rate resulting in secondary damage (this is explained on page 287); it also produces vasodilation, increasing the risk of bleeding and swelling. Cold therapy is used in the initial stages. Heat must *NOT* be given at any time, if there is extensive bruising or any risk of bleeding.

6 Mild heat can be applied in the subacute stage to promote healing of any condition which would benefit from increased metabolic rate, and increased blood supply. A greater range of movement may be possible after mild heating of the tissues due to increased flexibility.

Contra-indications to infra red treatments

1 Areas of defective skin sensation and hyper sensitive skin.
2 Recent scar tissue (defective sensitivity).
3 Extensive bruising or any area where there is a risk of bleeding.
4 Any undiagnosed injuries.
5 Skin disorders and diseases.
6 Heart conditions and blood pressure disorders (high or low).
7 Thrombosis or phlebitis or any areas of deficient circulation.
8 Recent exposure to UVL – sunburn.
9 Heavy colds and fevers.
10 Migraines and headaches.
11 Diabetes, as skin sensitivity may be impaired.
12 Any area where liniments or ointments have been applied.

Dangers of infra red treatments

1 Burns may be caused:
  A if heat is too intense
  B if the client is too near the lamp and fails to report overheating
  C if the skin sensation is defective and client may not be aware of overheating
  D if the client touches the lamp
  E if the lamp should fall and touch the client, or the bedding; overheating of pillows and blankets can cause fire and burns.
2 Electric shock – from faulty apparatus or water on treatment area producing short circuit.
3 Headache – irradiating the back of the neck and head, or over-heating by prolonged exposure may cause headache.
4 Faintness – over-heating or extensive irradiation may cause fall in blood pressure which may cause faintness.
5 Damage to eyes – IR exposure of the eyes can cause cataract. Clients should close the eyes and turn away from the lamp, wear goggles or have cotton wool over eyes.

Precautions to be taken when giving infra red treatment

1 Clean the skin with cologne or wash to remove sebum.
2 Ensure safe distance of the lamp from client. This distance depends on the client's tolerance and the output of the lamp (18–36 inches, 45–90 cms).
3 Do not place the lamp directly over client.
4 Ensure that lamp is stable, with the head over a foot if lamp has three or five feet.
5 Ensure that the lamp is in good working order and that there are no dents in the reflector.
6 Ensure that the flexes are sound and not trailing in a walking area.
7 Check for contra-indications.
8 Carry out a hot and cold sensitivity test.
9 Protect the eyes.
10 Explain the importance of calling immediately if the client feels too hot.
11 Warn the client not to move nearer to nor touch the lamp.

Treatment technique

Preparation of client

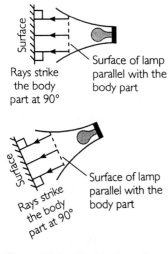

Rays strike the body part at 90°

Surface of lamp parallel with the body part

Rays strike the body part at 90°

Surface of lamp parallel with the body part

Figure 17.6 *Positioning of the lamp*

1 Place the client in a comfortable position. (When treating areas of the back, use side lying or recovery position, well supported by pillows. If treating knees or ankles, use half lying with pillows supporting the part. If treating the shoulders or the elbows, the client should be seated on a stool with the arms supported on a pillow.)
2 Check that all jewellery or metal has been removed from the area.
3 Uncover the area; wipe over with cleansing wipes.
4 Check for contra-indications.
5 Explain the treatment to the client; warn him/her not to touch the lamp.
6 Carry out a skin sensitivity test using two test tubes, one filled with hot water the other with cold water. Instruct the client to close her eyes. Touch the client with the hot test tube or the cold test tube, at random over the area. Ask the client if s/he feels hot or cold. (If the client cannot tell the difference between hot and cold, s/he has

defective sensation and the treatment should not be carried out.) Carry out the test all over the area to be irradiated.

7 Cover the areas not receiving treatment.

8 Warn the client that warmth should be mild and comfortable, and to call if the heat becomes too intense.

Procedure

1 Check plug, leads and reflector.

2 Switch lamp on, directed towards floor:
   A IR takes 10–15 minutes to reach maximum output.
   B Radiant heat (visible) takes around 2 minutes.

3 When maximum intensity is reached, position lamp, ensuring stability. (If lamp has 3 feet, place head of lamp over one of the feet, ensuring angle joints are secure.)

4 Make sure that the face of the lamp is parallel with the part so that the rays strike the part at 90° for maximum penetration, absorption and effect. Do not place the lamp directly above the client, in case the lamp drops or the bulb shatters.

5 Select an appropriate distance, between 45–90 cm (18–36 inches). The selected distance depends on two factors:
   A the intensity of the lamp
   B the client's tolerance.
   60 cm or 24 inches is a good average.

6 Ensure that the rays are not irradiating the client's eyes or face, or your own.

7 Observe the client throughout the treatment.

8 Treatment time: 20–30 minutes until desired effect is obtained. The client should not rise suddenly after IR treatment, because the blood pressure is lowered and s/he may feel faint.

9 The treatment may be followed by massage, warm up, stretch exercises or electrical treatments.

Heat treatment following injury

Heat treatment should not be given in the acute stage of injury because the increased metabolic rate and vasodilation (increasing blood flow and swelling) produced by heat will increase the extent of the injury rather than reduce it. Heat must not be used if there is any risk of bleeding either from open wounds or internally among the tissues.

Cold therapy should always be used initially because it decreases metabolic rate, produces vasoconstriction which will reduce bleeding, bruising and swelling, and also numbs the area which reduces pain.

After 72 hours or so, heat treatment can be given providing there is no further risk of bleeding. If there is extensive bruising, heat must not be given until healing is well under way and the bruise turns yellow. This may take six to twelve days.

Questions

1 List the contra-indications to heat therapy.
2 Give four differences between luminous and non luminous heat lamps.
3 Discuss the three factors which affect the intensity of radiation.
4 State the law that governs intensity in relation to distance.
5 Explain the effects of heat therapy.
6 Give four uses of heat treatment.
7 Explain why you would use heat therapy as a pre event treatment.

8 Explain why you would use heat therapy as a post event treatment.
9 Discuss the precautions to be taken when giving infra red treatment.
10 Explain how you would carry out a skin sensitivity test prior to infra red treatment.
11 Give the two factors which determine the distance of the lamp from the part.
12 Give the average time of infra red treatment.

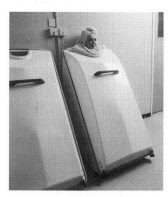

Figure 17.7 *A steam bath in use*

Steam treatments

This is used for general body heating. Steam may be applied to the body using steam baths or steam rooms. Steam treatments are used by athletes and sportspeople to promote relaxation, for deep cleansing and to make the tissues more receptive to any following treatments such as electrical muscle stimulation.

The steam bath

This bath is designed for individual treatments. It is a cabinet made of moulded fibreglass, in which the client sits.

It contains a trough with a heating element; water poured into the trough is heated, making steam. The trough is placed underneath an adjustable seat which allows the client to sit comfortably with the head outside the bath. There are usually three controls – a main switch, a timer and temperature gauge. The steam condenses within the bath, and the air is saturated with very high humidity of around 95%.

The steam room

This is a room which is supplied with steam from a boiler. Several people may use the steam room together. Some complexes based on Turkish baths have several rooms with increasing temperatures. Clients start with the lowest temperature and progress through to the highest.

The steam bath has several advantages over the steam room. However, group treatments in steam rooms are more sociable occasions.

Advantages of steam bath over steam room

1 The client does not feel claustrophobic because the head is out of the bath.
2 The client breathes normal air and not steam.
3 Hair remains neat and tidy and does not get wet.
4 The bath offers privacy for the client.
5 The temperature can be adjusted to suit the individual.
6 The initial cost and the running cost is low, compared with a steam room.
7 The bath takes up little space and can be accommodated in most clinics.

Effects of steam heat

1 A general rise in body temperature.
2 Increase in circulation due to vasodilation, giving hyperaemia and erythema.
3 Heart/pulse rate increases.
4 A fall in blood pressure due to dilation of superficial capillaries.
5 Increase in cell metabolism.

6 Stimulation of sweat glands with increased sweating and elimination of waste. There may be a temporary loss of body fluid due to sweating, but this is soon adjusted by drinking water.

7 Increased circulation and rise in temperature promotes muscle relaxation, reducing pain and stiffness.

8 Mild heat soothes sensory nerve endings.

Uses

- To prepare client for further treatment. Heating of the tissues prior to other treatments such as EMS or massage will increase their effectiveness.
- To induce relaxation and relieve pain and stiffness. This is particularly useful after training or performance.
- For deep cleansing, as sweating increases the elimination of waste.

Contra-indications

1 Heart and circulatory conditions.
2 High or low blood pressure.
3 Thrombosis and phlebitis.
4 Headaches, migraines, dizziness, faintness.
5 Skin diseases.
6 Athletes foot and verrucas.
7 Diabetics, epileptics.
8 Any chest conditions – asthmatics, bronchitis.
9 First days of menstruation.
10 Pregnancy.
11 After a heavy meal or drinking alcohol.
12 Client on a low calorie slimming diet.

Dangers

1 Over-heating causing fainting or dizziness.
2 Burns from touching hot metal trough.
3 Cross infection of micro-organisms.

Precautions

1 Ensure good standards of hygiene, as moist heat is an ideal breeding ground for micro-organisms. Wipe over the whole bath with sterilising detergent before and after treatment. Cover the seat and floor with towels which are boiled after use or disposed of.
2 Check that the power supply and terminals are correctly switched on.
3 Check that the trough is full of *distilled* water which will prevent scaling around the element.
4 Protect the client from direct contact with metal and steam, using a towel.
5 Remove jewellery, glasses, contact lenses etc.
6 Check for contra-indications – examine the feet for athlete's foot and verrucas.
7 Ensure that the client takes a shower before treatment to remove any oils, linaments, etc., and also after treatment.
8 Use disposable slippers and paper on the floor.
9 Explain treatment to client and demonstrate how to open the door and get out of the bath.
10 Wrap a towel around neck to prevent steam escaping.
11 Stay within calling distance of client and observe frequently.

Treatment technique

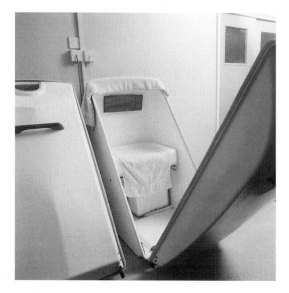

Figure 17.8 *Preparation of a steam bath*

Preparation of bath before client arrives

1 Wipe over with sterilising detergent.
2 Fill the trough with distilled water.
3 Protect the seat with a towel and ensure that the client is protected from contact with metal or direct steam.
4 Place a towel over the aperture to prevent loss of steam.
5 Turn on the main switch and bath switch.
6 Turn the controls to maximum until the water is heating, and then adjust the temperature and timer (50°C–55°C). The bath will take around 15 minutes to heat from cold.

Procedure

1 Supply client with gown and paper slippers.
2 Remove all jewellery, glasses, contact lenses etc.
3 Check for contra-indications.
4 Explain the treatment to the client and show how to enter and leave the steam bath/room.
5 Help client into shower.
6 After shower help client into bath, make sure that s/he is comfortable, close the door.
7 Place towel around client's neck over the aperture.
8 Keep in verbal contact throughout; be reassuring and ask the client to report any discomfort.
9 Treatment time is 15–20 minutes.
10 Help client from bath and into shower.
11 The client may use a friction rub to improve skin texture.
12 Client should now rest for 20–30 minutes or receive further treatments but *not exercise.*

Sauna Baths

These baths are pine wood log cabins heated by electric stoves. They are manufactured in various sizes, from a single person sauna up to large cabins for 10–14 people. In Scandinavian countries they are found indoor and outdoor. The larger the sauna, the more expensive it will be to run, as it will require more heat output from larger stoves.

The walls of the cabin are constructed of well insulated panels of pine wood. Pine wood allows interchange of air and absorbs moisture. This will reduce the humidity inside the cabin, giving a dry heat. The heat is provided by electric

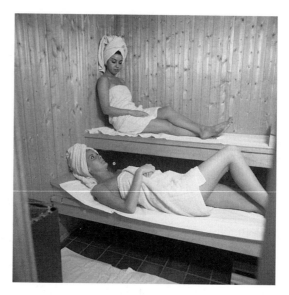

Figure 17.9   *A sauna bath*

stoves which heat non-splintering stones placed on top of
the stove. Slatted wooden benches are arranged inside the
sauna for sitting or lying down. There is an air inlet near
the floor and an outlet near the ceiling. As the air in the
sauna is heated, it rises by convection, therefore the sauna is
hotter on the upper benches than on the lower benches.

The air moisture is absorbed by the walls, making
humidity very low (around 10%). This humidity can easily
be increased by pouring water on the stones which boils,
making steam. Creating steam makes the body hotter.
Because the humidity in the sauna is low, sweat from the
body evaporates quickly and cools the body; therefore, high
temperatures can be tolerated in the sauna. The
temperature in the sauna may range from 50°C to around
120°C.

A temperature range between 60°C to 80°C is
recommended for clients unfamiliar with sauna baths. This
can be increased as the client's tolerance increases. The
thermometer should always be checked for the temperature
and the hygrometer should be checked for humidity before
commencement of treatment. These are found on a wall
inside the cabin. Humidity range from 50% to 70% is most
comfortable.

Uses

- Mainly used after training or performance to reduce pain and stiffness.
- To induce relaxation.
- For deep cleansing.

Effects

1 General rise in body temperature.
2 Increase in circulation.
3 Heart rate increases.
4 Superficial capillaries dilate, therefore fall in blood pressure.
5 Erythema produced.
6 Increase in cell metabolism.
7 Increased sweating with elimination of waste.
8 Produces relaxation, relieves pain and stiffness.
9 Sedatory effect on nerve endings.
10 If sweating is excessive, can produce dehydration.
11 The dry heat is irritating and drying to mucous membranes.

Contra-indications

1 Heart and circulatory conditions.
2 High and low blood pressure.
3 Thrombosis, phlebitis.
4 Headaches, dizziness, migraines, faintness.
5 Skin diseases.
6 Athlete's foot, verrucas.
7 Diabetics, epileptics.
8 Chest conditions – asthmatics, bronchitis.
9 First days of menstruation.
10 Pregnancy.
11 After heavy meals or alcohol.
12 Clients on low calorie diets.

Dangers

1 Fainting or dizziness if blood pressure falls too low.
2 Dehydration with prolonged and frequent treatments.

3 Dryness and irritation of mucous membranes, eg, throat, nose etc.

The therapist should always supervise the sauna.

Precautions

1 Check temperature and humidity before use (temp. 60°C–80°C, humidity 50–70% is most comfortable).
2 Check that the guard around heating element is secure and in position.
3 The client must shower to remove any oils, linaments, make up, etc.
4 Ensure client removes contact lenses, glasses and jewellery.
5 Examine the client for contra-indications, particularly the feet for athlete's foot and verrucas.
6 Use disposable slippers and paper on floor.
7 Observe client throughout treatment and check time.
8 Boil towels or robes after each treatment.
9 Scrub benches and floor thoroughly with sterilising fluid after use.

Treatment technique

1 Prepare the sauna before client arrives. Protect the floor with paper towelling and bench with towels.
2 Explain the procedure to the client and stress that she must come out if she feels dizzy or faint.
3 Client should shower before treatment.
4 Client should wear some form of hair protection.
5 Client enters the sauna with or without towel wrap and wears disposable slippers.
6 Advise the client to sit or lie on the lower benches until accustomed to the heat (hot air rises therefore lower benches are at lower temperature).
7 Small amounts of water may be sprinkled on the stones from time to time to increase humidity (this should not be overdone).
8 Treatment time will depend on tolerance of client. First treatment could be up to 5 minutes, increasing to 14 minutes or 20 minutes as tolerance is built up.

9 Warm or cold showers may be taken during the course of the treatment.
10 The client must always shower after sauna.
11 Rest after treatment or continue with other treatments such as massage, but *no exercise.*
12 Scrub benches and floor thoroughly with sterilising fluid.

Differences between steam baths and saunas

	Steam	Sauna
1	Moist heat, humidity 95%	Dry heat, humidity 10%
2	Atmospheric air is inhaled therefore more suitable for clients with mild respiratory problems.	Hot dry air is inhaled which may irritate the mucous membranes.
3	Easily adjusted to the tolerance of individual clients.	Usually communal, therefore difficult to adjust to the needs of individual clients.
4	Not claustrophobic as head is free.	May be claustrophobic.
5	Not as damaging to hair which remains outside the bath.	May damage hair particularly permed or coloured hair.
6	Ensures privacy of client.	Lacks privacy if communal.
7	Inexpensive to run but may be less profitable as only one client can be treated.	Expensive to run but may be more profitable as many clients may be treated at one time.
8	Comfortable for most clients.	Less comfortable for the older less mobile clients or those with sensitive skins.

Spa pools/baths

These refer to baths for sitting in rather than swimming. They vary in size and construction, from preformed, reinforced acrylic shells to block-built and tiled baths. Spa baths contain a quantity of water which is heated, chemically treated and filtered. Hydrojet circulation and air induction bubbles may also be included.

A spa bath is not drained, cleaned and refilled after each individual user, as a whirlpool bath would be. Cleaning and water change is only carried out after a specific number of people have used the bath. The frequency of water change will depend on the capacity of the bath and the number of users.

Spas may be classified into residential spas or commercial spas. Residential spas are installed for private use in the home, while commercial spas are installed for general use in premises such as hotels, health clubs, sports centres, gymnasia, salons and clinics.

Installation of spa baths

Spas must be installed by experienced contractors in accordance with the Swimming Pool and Allied Trades Association (SPATA) standards. The spa must be installed on a level solid base; if the spa is to be installed on a suspended floor, consideration must be given to the weight of the bath plus water and bathers. The contractor must ensure that the support is adequate.

All spa equipment must be properly installed and connected; all components must be accessible for maintenance. The spa must be positioned so that any noise will not cause undue disturbance. Ventilation in the area of the spa should be adequate to prevent condensation.

All surfaces must be smooth, with rounded moulded edges. Uneven surfaces or sharp edges may cause accidents and injuries. The wet floor area around the spa should have a non-porous, non-slip, even surface, and must be easy to clean and sanitise. There must be adequate drainage to ensure that water spillage flows away quickly.

The contractor must ensure that the water provided to fill the spa is of satisfactory quality. If the water supply does not meet the required standards, steps must be taken to bring the water within chemical, physical and biological standards.

The contractor must advise and instruct the operator on the operational procedures required and the treatments necessary to maintain water quality and to achieve the highest standards of hygiene and safety. Advice must also be given on the correct handling and safe storage of chemicals. A manual listing all these instructions must be provided by the manufacturer or constructor and explained to the operator. The contractor must also supply a water testing kit and explain its use and limitations.

Guidelines for water standards

The source of water for the spa pool is usually from the main supply. If this is not available, water may be obtained from other sources which must be assessed and deemed suitable by a public analyst. After treatment the water should be within the following standards:

- disinfectant levels: a bromine residual of 4–6 mg/litre for commercial spas, 2–4 mg/litre for residential spas.
- a free chlorine residual of 3–5 mg/litre for commercial spas, 1.5–3 mg/litre for residential spas. Ozone may be used in conjunction with bromine and chlorine.
- pH levels: 7.2–7.8
- total alkalinity: 80–160/mg/litre as calcium carbonate
- calcium hardness: 75–500 mg/litre as calcium carbonate
- total dissolved solids: less than 1500 mg/litre

Proper standards of disinfection must be maintained at all times. The environmental health officer for the local authority will carry out a routine assessment of the biological purity of the spa water. The recommendation for spa water is as follows:

- to contain less than 100 bacteria per ml capable of growing on agar in two days at 37°C.
- to be free from Coliforms, Pseudomonas, Staphylococcus and Faecal Streptococcus in 100 ml water.

Purification

Organic and nitrogenous impurities are introduced into the spa water during normal use, therefore filtration and chemical treatment is essential to remove and break down this matter and to purify the recycled water. Algae growths may occur in some spas, and while these are not generally harmful to health, they make surfaces slippery and make the water look unattractive. A number of spa disinfectants are effective in limiting these growths, but if necessary, recommended algicides may be used. Foaming may occur as a result of soap being introduced into the spa after users have showered. This can be removed using an anti-foam agent.

Additional chemicals

In addition to the chemicals discussed above, other chemical products may be required to maintain water standards as listed below:

1 Aluminium sulphate – to aid filtration
2 Calcium chloride – to raise calcium hardness
3 Polyelectrolyte products – to aid filtration
4 Sodium bicarbonate – to raise total alkalinity
5 Sodium carbonate (soda ash) – to raise pH
6 Sodium hydrogen sulphate – to lower pH
7 Sodium thiosulphate – to dechlorinate and debrominate water
8 Sequestering agents – to protect against staining and scale formation

Use of spa pools

■ To promote relaxation.
■ To relieve muscular aches and pains.
■ To ease joint pain and stiffness.

Effects

1 An increase in the circulation.
2 An increase in heart/pulse rate.
3 A fall in blood pressure as the superficial blood vessels dilate.
4 A rise in body temperature.
5 The warmth induces muscle relaxation.
6 Soothing of sensory nerve endings.
7 An increase in cell metabolism due to warmth and increased circulation.
8 Increased pressure near the jets has an invigorating effect.

Contra-indications

These should be displayed near the pool and must be explained to each client. Clients must seek medical advice before using the spa if any of the following conditions apply:

1 Heart disease or circulatory conditions such as high or low blood pressure.
2 A history of thrombosis, embolism or phlebitis.
3 Pregnancy.
4 Chest conditions such as asthma and bronchitis.
5 Epilepsy or diabetes.
6 Undiagnosed swellings.
7 If taking medication.
8 Following recent operation.

Do not use the spa if you are suffering any of the following:

■ headache, migraine, faintness, dizziness, fever
■ any infections such as colds or flu etc
■ skin diseases or infections
■ extensive bruising or any history of haemorrhage
■ cuts and abrasions
■ athletes foot or verruca
■ after eating a meal or drinking alcohol
■ if on a low calorie diet.

Dangers in the use of spa pools

1 Nausea, faintness, dizziness or headache may result from over use. Limit the time spent in the spa to 10–20 minutes.
2 Cross infection of micro-organisms.
3 Skin irritation caused by the chemicals in the water.
4 Slipping or falling if the pool surround is wet and slippery.

Precautions

■ Tell the person in charge if you are to be alone in the bath.
■ Children must not use the bath without supervision.

- Shower before and after using the bath.
- Do not stay in the bath for too long: 10–20 minutes only.
- Come out if feeling too hot, faint, nauseous or dizzy.
- Enter the bath and exit slowly holding on to the safety rail.
- Do not enter the bath if it already contains the recommended number of bathers.
- Check the spa temperature before use, the maximum safe temperature is 40°C (104°F).
- Do not sit directly in front of the jets.
- Shower after bathing, to cool down.

Operation and care of spa pool/bath

Those responsible for the operation and care of spa pools, must be familiar with and operate according to the legislation and codes of practice related to spa pools. Copies of these documents should be available at all times and studied in detail. These include:

1 Health and Safety at Work Act 1974
2 Safety in Swimming Pools – Health and Safety Commissions and Sports Council
3 The Swimming Pool and Allied Trades Association (SPATA) Guidelines
4 Code of Practice For Hygiene in Beauty Salons and Clinics

The highest standards of hygiene and safety must be practised at all times. Every precaution must be taken to avoid cross infection or injury to the client.

Operator responsibilities

Spa baths differ in size, construction and in mode of operation. It is therefore important that each operator is fully conversant with all the detail in the manufacturer's instruction manual for their particular spa. This must be obtained from the manufacturer or contractor when the bath is installed. It is the contractor's duty to explain and discuss the procedures with the operator and to give advice as required.

The operator must carry out the following procedures in accordance with the manufacturers instructions:

1 Fill the bath to the correct level with water and ensure that this level is maintained

2 Ensure that the pump, filter and any other devices are working correctly and are regularly cleaned and maintained.

3 Maintain the correct disinfection levels in the bath at all times; chlorine or bromine are generally added to the water either manually or automatically. It is recommended that a bromine residual of 4–6 mg/litre should be maintained in the water of a commercial spa or a chlorine residual of 3–5 mg/litre. Excess of these chemicals may cause skin irritation and smarting of the eyes.

4 Maintain the correct pH levels in the bath at all times. 7.2–7.8 is the recommended range, 7.4–7.6 is the ideal. The correct pH level is important to prevent corrosion and scale formation, and for effective disinfection and client comfort. All commercial spas should have automatic controllers to provide continuous monitoring and control of disinfectant and pH levels.

5 Clean the water line regularly with the recommended non-foaming cleaner. This improves the hygiene standards and the appearance of the bath.

6 Remove any foam which may occur with an anti-foaming agent as this affects the clarity of the water.

7 Add a sequestering agent at the first sign of staining or scale formation which will be unattractive and may cause corrosion and block pipework.

8 Maintain a water temperature of 38°C. The water temperature must not exceed the maximum recommended temperature of 40°C.

9 Change the water, clean the bath and its equipment regularly. The frequency of this operation will depend on the size and usage of the bath. A daily change may be required for heavily used commercial baths. The current guideline indicates that the water should be changed when the number of users has equalled one half of the spa water capacity; eg, for a bath containing 660 gallons of water, 330 bathers may use the bath before a change of water is required. Clean the bath with a recommended cleaning agent before refilling.

10 Test the chemical levels regularly according to the manufacturers instructions.
Note: Chemicals must not be mixed with each other, either in a dry state or in solution. All chemicals must be

added to the spa water as indicated in the instruction manual, either directly or via a chemical feeder.

11 Record all tests, changes and any maintenance work undertaken. For every chemical test, the time, result and action taken must be recorded in a record book or chart. This must be accessible to all operators. An instrument to continuously record disinfectant and pH levels is strongly recommended.

12 Keep detailed client records, which should include usage of the bath.

13 Ensure that bathers are seated correctly in the pool. They must be observed at all times, and should they become unwell, assist them carefully out of the pool.

14 Ensure that the number of bathers in the pool at any one time does not exceed the number recommended for that pool.

15 Rowdy behaviour must not be allowed in the spa. Such behaviour must be dealt with quickly, politely but firmly. All those involved should be asked to refrain from such behaviour or told to leave the pool. Help should be sought from colleagues, supervisors or managers if the situation becomes difficult.

16 Take particular care with the handling and storage of chemicals. Read and follow the guidelines on the packages. Be aware of the legislative requirements regarding these products.

17 Operators must be up to date with any new guidelines and legislative requirements relating to spa pools and chemical products.

Protection of the operator

For the protection and safety of the operator, the following protective clothing should be worn when handling chemicals:

- apron: a bib type apron in pvc
- gloves: waterproof
- goggles: chemical BSI standard
- respirator mask: recommended type
- a First Aid box with an eye wash bottle should be kept near the spa bath.

Preparation of the client

1 Greet in client in a pleasant manner and reassure him/her.
2 Complete a record card.
3 Check for contra-indications and explain these to the client. Seek medical advice where there is uncertainty.
4 Conduct the client to the changing room and explain the procedure.
5 Give the client a robe and towel.
6 Ask the client to remove jewellery, glasses, contact lenses, change into his/her swimsuit and cover the hair if desired.
7 Explain the importance of taking a shower before entering the bath, for reasons of hygiene, and to remove any oils, lotions, make up or perfume. Ask the client to rinse thoroughly to remove all traces of soap as any residue may affect the chemical balance of the water and produce foaming if carried into the bath.
8 Conduct the client to the bath and show him/her where to enter.
9 Advise the client to sit between the jets.
10 Tell the client that the recommended time in the bath is 10–20 minutes (maximum time is 20 minutes). The client should come out immediately if he/she feels unwell, dizzy or weak.
11 Observe the spa at all times when in use, give assistance as required.
12 Explain the importance of taking a shower after the bath to cool down and wash off any residue. Advise the client to dry thoroughly and moisturise the skin. The client should then rest or receive further treatment such as massage.

Paraffin wax

Paraffin wax treatment can be used for the whole body, for the hands and feet or for muscle strains of the legs and arms. Wax is messy and difficult to apply to certain areas; other forms of heat are easier to use.

Equipment

When cold, the wax is whitish and solid, but when heated it liquefies and clarifies.

Wax is heated in containers, which vary in size and shape. The larger models have a water jacket and automatic temperature controls. Wax is heated and maintained at a temperature of 45–49°C. The warm wax is applied in layers, using a brush or ladle. When treating hands and feet, these can be quickly dipped into the wax. Each layer of wax is allowed to dry and become white before the next coat is applied. A build up of six coats is desirable. The area is then wrapped in polythene, grease proof paper or tinfoil and covered with a towel to retain the heat.

The application of wax can be messy and care must be taken to cover the floor and clothing before the treatment starts.

The application of wax to body parts – uses

1 To relieve pain and stiffness of injured joints.
2 To promote relaxation of muscles.
3 To increase the extensibility of ligaments and tendons.
4 To increase the circulation and promote healing.
5 To decrease stiffness in arthritic joints. Exercises given after wax may result in increased mobility.

Effects

1 The heat raises the temperature of the area. This promotes relaxation and relieves pain and stiffness.
2 Heat reduces tension and improves the extensibility of muscles.
3 There is an increase in circulation due to vasodilation, giving hyperaemia and erythema. This speeds up the healing processes.
4 The heat soothes sensory nerve endings relieving pain.
5 Stimulation of sweat glands and more sweat is produced.
6 Stimulation of sebaceous glands and the grease in the wax softens the skin.
7 Increases the flexibility of ligaments and tendons.
8 Increase in metabolic rate.

Contra-indications

1 Skin diseases and disorders, particularly verrucae, athlete's foot and eczema.
2 Cuts and abrasions; small cuts can be covered with waterproof plaster.
3 Severe bruising or swelling or any risk of bleeding.
4 Any skin infections.
5 Undiagnosed painful areas; seek medical advice.
6 Very hairy areas.

Dangers

Burns of the skin if the temperature is too high – 49°C is the correct temperature. (Use a sugar thermometer if the wax bath is not automatically controlled.)

Precautions

1 Cover all areas not receiving treatment.
2 Test the wax on self before treatment.
3 Do not hold the part in the wax bath.
4 Lay a towel then greaseproof paper or foil under the part.

Treatment technique

Preparation of client

1 Place the client in a well supported comfortable position.
2 Check that all clothing or jewellery in the area has been removed.
3 Check for contra-indications.
4 Cover the floor and protect client's clothing.
5 Wash the area thoroughly with warm soapy water, rinse and dry.
6 Explain the procedure to the client.

Procedure

1 Check the temperature of the wax on self and on the client.
2 Hold the part above the bath if possible, or over a bowl or paper to catch surplus wax. Apply a thin coat of wax

with brush or ladle and allow to dry. Repeat five or six times until the part is well covered. Work quickly.

3 Cover with polythene, grease proof paper or tinfoil and then wrap in a towel.

4 Leave the wax on for around 20 minutes.

5 Remove the towel and paper and slide off the wax.

6 Pat the area with a tissue to dry.

7 Dispose of wax into a boiler or into a bin.

8 Follow with other treatments.

Care and maintenance of wax

Wax is supplied as large blocks, which should be covered and kept in a dry cupboard. Check the blocks before placing in the bath; remove any dirt, hairs etc. After use, the wax may be disposed of by wrapping in paper and placing in a bin. However this proves expensive and the wax may be re-used if it is cleaned and sterilised.

To clean the wax, take a large metal bowl and pour in two to three pints of water. Put all the used wax into the bowl. At the end of the day, place the bowl on a heating plate and bring to the boil. Boil for over 20 minutes then turn off heat. Leave overnight; the wax will rise to the top and solidify, and the water and other matter will remain underneath. Prise out the wax and scrape all debris from the underside. It may be necessary to remove a quarter to a half inch of the wax. When the wax is clean again, it can be re-used in the wax bath.

Throw away the water and debris in the bowl and wash the bowl thoroughly with hot soapy water.

Questions

1 Explain why hyperaemia and erythema occur as a result of heat on the tissues.

2 State what happens to the following when the body is heated:
   A The heart and pulse rate.
   B The blood pressure.

3 Give six advantages of using a steam bath rather than steam room.

4 Give the temperatures recommended for the following treatments:
   A Steam bath
   B Sauna

C Wax application.

5 Give three dangers associated with sauna treatments.

6 Explain the procedure for preparing the sauna and the client before sauna treatment.

7 List ten contra-indications to steam treatment.

8 Explain the precautions to be taken before the application of wax treatments.

CHAPTER 18

Mechanical Massage

Mechanical massage is the manipulation of body tissues using machines. It is generally used in conjunction with other treatments to relieve muscle tension and muscle pain, improve the blood circulation and lymphatic drainage, and improve the condition of certain skin types. The use of machines provides a deep and vigorous treatment and is not as tiring for the therapist. Various types of massage appliances are manufactured, from the small hand held percussion and audio-sonic equipment designed to treat small, localised areas, to the large and heavy gyratory vibrators used for deeper effects on larger areas of the body.

Mechanical massage for sports therapy

The effects of mechanical massage are similar to those of manual massage, but the sensation felt by the client is very different. The treatment is rather impersonal and the use of a machine rather than the touch of hands is not as pleasing to the client. In sports therapy, mechanical vibratory treatments should be combined with some manual massage, thus gaining the more personal aspects of manual massage combined with the depth and power of vibratory equipment.

Mechanical massage is usually used where additional depth is required as it is less tiring for the therapist when a long, vigorous manual massage is required. The smaller head of the audio-sonic vibrator is useful on small areas, particularly around joints and over fibrositic or tension nodules. The effects produced are similar for all types of massage equipment, but are deeper and greater with the heavier machines. The treatment is very popular with clients as it feels invigorating and they feel that desired results will be achieved.

There are three types of mechanical massage equipment:

1 Gyratory vibrators – floor standing models.
2 Gyratory vibrators – hand held.
3 Audio-sonic – hand held massager.

The gyratory vibrator

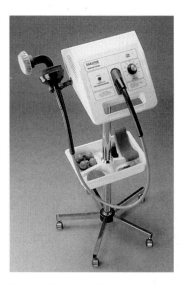

Figure 18.1   *A floor standing gyratory vibrator*

Massage with this type of appliance is much heavier than with audio-sonic vibrators. It is therefore more suitable for heavier work on large and bulky areas of the body. There are two main types of appliance:

1 *The hand held vibrator:* this is heavy and cumbersome to use, as all the electrical component parts are held in the hand. However it is portable and useful for work outside the clinic.
2 *The floor standing gyratory vibrator (commonly called G5):* this is a very useful treatment in the clinic. All the electrical components are housed in a box which is supported by a stand, and only the moving head is held in the hand. This machine uses a rotary electric motor to turn a crank which is attached to the head. The head turns in gyratory motion, moving round and round, up and down and side to side with pressure, providing a deep massage. A variety of attachments are available which screw onto the head. They are designed to simulate the movements of manual massage:
   A Effleurage: sponge heads, curved and disc.
   B Petrissage: hard rubber heads, flat disc, four half ball (egg box), multi-hard spike.
   C Tapotement: fine spiky and brush heads.

Uses

1 *Pre-event:* to warm up muscles prior to performance. It may be used after heating the tissues, and combined with manual massage over the muscles and joints involved in the activities. It must be used for a short time only, five minutes or so. Follow with the warm up exercise routine.

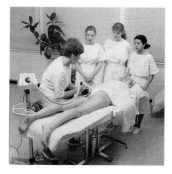

Figure 18.2 *Demonstration of treatment using gyratory massager*

The treatment should not be used for the first time on the day of an event. The athlete must be familiar with its use during training sessions as the rate and depth must be selected to suit the individual; it is important that it does not interfere with his timing and rhythm.

2 *Post event:* to hasten muscle recovery following performance and cool down. Great care must be taken if using mechanical massage following a performance, as there may be tissue injury which is not immediately obvious. It is far better to use hand massage, as any tension in the tissues will be felt and the pressure adjusted accordingly. If there is little tension and no pain, light mechanical massage with light pressure may follow.

3 To generally relieve muscular tension and reduce muscular aches and pains.

4 To improve poor circulation and speed up venous drainage.

5 To improve the circulation around joints, increasing warmth and improving the flexibility of ligaments (use the sponge head only).

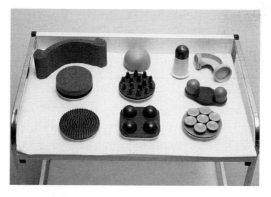

Figure 18.3 *Different heads for the gyratory massager*

Effects

1 As with manual massage, the main effect is stimulation of the circulation. The movements speed up the flow of blood in the veins, removing de-oxygenated blood and waste products more rapidly. As the venous flow speeds up, so does the arterial circulation, bringing warm

oxygenated blood and nutrients to the area.

2 The increased blood supply and friction of the heads will raise the temperature of the area. This warmth will improve muscle elasticity, contractability and the flexibility of tendons and ligaments.

3 The increased blood flow will speed up the removal of waste products such as lactic acid, which accumulate in the muscles following intense activity. This will hasten muscle recovery, promote relaxation and relieve pain and stiffness.

4 The increased delivery of nutrients and oxygen will increase the metabolic rate in the tissues. This will improve the condition of the tissues and aid their recovery.

5 Lymph drainage via the lymphatic vessels is also increased, which also aids the removal of waste products and fluid from the tissue spaces.

6 Surface capillaries dilate, producing an erythema; the desquamating effect of the heads will improve texture of the skin.

Contra-indications

1 Skin infections, diseases or disorders, any large skin tags, warts or pigmented moles.

2 Any acute tissue injury such as sprains, strains, tears, bruising; any risk of bleeding.

3 Dilated capillaries or over varicose veins.

4 On spastic (hypertoned) or on flaccid (hypotoned) muscles.

5 Thrombosis or phlebitis.

6 Recent fractures.

7 Recent operations and scar tissue.

8 Treatment of abdomen during pregnancy and menstruation.

9 Extremely hairy areas.

10 Thin, bony clients.

11 Elderly clients with thin crêpy skin and lack of subcutaneous fat.

12 Acute back and spinal problems, eg, disc trouble.

Dangers

Heavy and prolonged treatments can cause bruising and dilated capillaries. If used too soon following injury, it may increase tissue damage.

Precautions

1 Check for contra-indications.
2 Do not use heavy percussion over bony areas, or over areas with poor muscle tone.
3 Do not over-treat one area; keep the massage head moving.
4 Keep the head surface parallel with the surface of the body, and adapt to body contours.
5 Hold the head away from the client when switching on, in case it is insecure and becomes detached. Hold below the couch for safety.
6 Cover the heads with a plastic bag, which can be changed for each client for hygienic reasons.

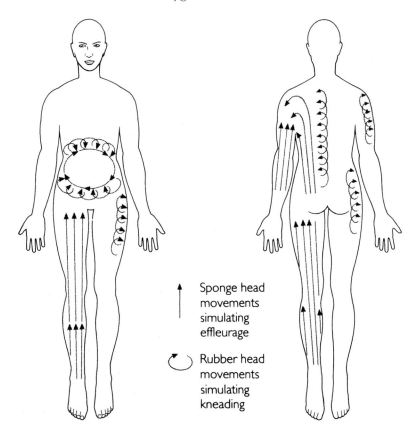

Sponge head movements simulating effleurage

Rubber head movements simulating kneading

Figure 18.4 *Direction of strokes for gyratory massager*

Treatment technique

Preparation of client

1 Place the client in a well supported, comfortable position.
2 Check that all clothing and jewellery has been removed from the area.
3 Check for contra-indications.
4 Clean the skin with cologne or skin cleanser such as savlon or soap and water.
5 Explain the treatment to the client.
6 Pre-heat the area if appropriate.
7 Apply talcum powder to the area using effleurage strokes (do not use oil as it may cause deterioration of the sponge heads, but check this with the manufacturer).

Procedure

1 Select the appropriate heads to suit the needs of the client. Do not change the heads too often as this breaks the continuity of the treatment:
   A For effleurage: curved sponge on limbs or round sponge around joints and elsewhere.
   B For kneading: the flat disk head for lighter petrissage; the four ball head for deeper petrissage; the multi large spike for very deep petrissage on very well toned muscle bulk or over heavy areas of adipose tissue.
   C For desquamating and surface erythema: fine spiky and brush heads.
   To maintain high standards of hygiene, the heads can be placed in a plastic bag which is changed for each client.
2 Switch the machine on, holding the head below the level of the couch. (This is a safety precaution in case the head is insecure; if it flies off it will not hit the client.)
3 With the sponge applicator, apply in long sweeping strokes following the direction of venous return and natural contours of the body. The stroke at make and break should be light and smooth rather than abrupt and jerky. The pressure should be heavier on muscle bulk. Cover the area well.
4 Change the head for kneading. Use circular kneading motion, using the other hand to support the tissues and lift them towards the head. Again apply upward pressure and work with venous return. Cover the area well.

5 Keep the surface of the attachment parallel with the surface of the body at all times. (If one side lifts off the body there is a danger of damaging the tissues with the hard edge of the head.)

6 Change to effleurage head to complete the treatment.

7 The degree of erythema and client tolerance dictates the length of the treatment.

8 Wash heads in hot water and detergent; allow to dry.

Note: Particular care should be taken when selecting heads for treating the abdominal wall. Abdominal organs have no bony framework for protection. In front their only protection is provided by the muscles and tissues of the abdominal wall. If these muscles are over-stretched with poor tone, they offer less protection. This must be considered when treating the abdomen. The heavier petrissage heads should only be used on well toned abdominal muscles with a covering of adipose tissue, eg, the very fit or younger overweight client.

Audio-sonic vibrator

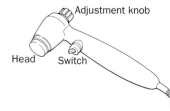

Figure 18.5 *Audio-sonic vibrator*

This is a hand held appliance. Its name is derived from audio (hearing) and sonic (sound); the humming sound produced by this machine can be heard (but it should not be confused with ultra-sound therapy, which is quite different). This uses an electro magnet. When the current is passing one way, the coil moves forward; as the current reverses, the coil moves back. This movement forward and backward is transmitted to the head of the appliance. When the head is placed on the tissues, the forward–backward movement of the coil alternately compresses and decompresses the tissues. Because the head does not physically move back and fore, this appliance has a gentle action. It penetrates quite deeply into the tissues but is not stimulating on the surface of the skin. It is particularly useful on small areas within muscles such as fibrositic nodules or areas of soreness and tension. It is also useful in the treatment of ligaments around joints. It may be fitted with different heads which usually include:

■ A flat head for larger surface massage.
■ A curved head for deeper work over tension or fibrositic nodules.

Uses

1 To relieve pain and stiffness in localised areas within muscles.
2 To produce warmth and aid relaxation of muscle fibres.
3 To stimulate the circulation around joints, thus improving flexibility.
4 To promote healing of chronic ligamentous sprains.
5 To break down fibrositic nodules within muscles.

Effects

1 Increase in the circulation to the localised area.
2 Dilation of superficial capillaries, producing an erythema.
3 Increase in the metabolic rate in the area, thus improving the condition of the tissues and aiding recovery.
4 Rise in the temperature producing warmth in the area which promotes relaxation of muscle fibres.
5 Increased warmth increases flexibility of ligaments around joints.

Contra-indications

1 Any skin infections, diseases or disorders in the area.
2 Dilated capillaries or over varicose veins.
3 Recent acute injury or healing tissues.
4 Over bruises or if there is any risk of bleeding in the area.
5 On spastic (hypertoned) or on flaccid (hypotoned) muscles.
6 Over skin tags, warts or unidentified pigmented area.

Treatment technique

Preparation of client

1 Place the client in a well supported and comfortable position.
2 Check that all clothing and jewellery has been removed from the area.
3 Check for contra-indications.

4 Explain the treatment to the client.
5 Cleanse the skin.
6 Apply talcum powder or cream to the skin. (Read the manufacturer's instruction, as some indicate that no medium should be used.)

Procedure

1 Select the appropriate head and secure firmly.
2 Switch machine on away from the client.
3 Commence the treatment using a circular motion; ensure good coverage of the area. Protect any prominent bony areas with the other hand.
4 The skin reaction indicates the length of the treatment time. When an even erythema is produced, the treatment should stop. This may take between 5–15 minutes.
5 Do not keep the vibrator on the same point – move it around in small circles.
6 Complete the treatment with manual stroking and effleurage to the area.
7 Remove the talcum or cream.
8 Clean the heads, wash with hot water and detergent and disinfect with surgical wipes.

Questions

1 Give three uses for mechanical massage on the body.
2 Name two different types of mechanical massage equipment.
3 List four contra-indications to mechanical massage on the body.
4 List the effects of mechanical massage on the body.
5 Explain briefly why the audio-sonic vibrator is used over tension nodules within muscles.
6 Give four effects of audio-sonic vibrator treatment.
7 Give two different uses for each of the following
   A Gyratory vibrator (G5).
   B Audio-sonic vibrator.
8 Explain briefly how you would incorporate mechanical massage into a post event treatment routine.
9 Give reasons why the heavy gyratory vibrator heads should not be used on the abdominal wall of certain clients.
10 Explain the procedure for maintaining high standards of hygiene when using gyratory vibrators.

CHAPTER 19

Muscle Stimulation

Electrical pulses produced by machines can be used to stimulate motor nerves which results in the contraction of muscles supplied by that nerve. Normal muscle contraction is controlled by the brain. Impulses initiated in the brain are transmitted via the spinal cord and the motor nerves to the muscles, stimulating their contraction. Pulses of current produced by machines and applied to the motor nerve by electrodes will produce the same result; ie, contraction of the muscles supplied by that nerve.

Indications for use

A variety of muscle stimulators are to be found on the market, ranging from simple single outlet machines with pre-set controls to the very complex machines with multi outlets and a range of variable controls. However they all produce electrical pulses which are applied to the body by means of electrodes.

The muscles are made to contract and relax, simulating active exercise. The treatment is used to improve muscle *tone* and condition and to maintain muscle *strength*. There is still considerable doubt as to whether electrical stimulation of normal muscle will produce a significant increase in muscle strength; voluntary progressively resisted exercises are essential for increasing muscle strength. However, electrical stimulation is very effective in re-educating muscle action following injury or periods of immobility. When muscles are weak, electrical stimulation combined with exercise is more effective in increasing strength than exercises alone. The use of electrical muscle stimulation, together with resisted exercise in the initial stages of training, is particularly effective, but as strength develops over three to four weeks, it may be phased out.

Terminology of muscle stimulation

The original current used for muscle stimulation was produced by the Smart-Bristow coil, and was known as the Faradic current. This term is sometimes used today to describe muscle stimulating treatments, eg, Faradism or Faradic treatment. The terms TENS, EMS and NMES (NMS) are also used.

- TENS – transcutaneous electrical nerve stimulation. This type of stimulation with low frequency current is used for pain control and is generally applied under medical supervision. Modern equipment may include TENS to reduce pain and therefore improve client comfort.
- EMS – electrical muscle stimulation. This term covers stimulation of both innervated muscle and denervated muscle (denervated muscle means one lacking in nerve supply due to injury or disease). Different types of pulses are used for these two forms.
- NMS/NMES – neuro-muscular (electrical) stimulation. This term covers the stimulation of innervated muscle. In sports therapy, stimulation will always be applied to normal muscle which will use nerve stimulation to produce muscle contraction. Therefore it is more accurate to use the term NMES or NMS when referring to these treatments. However, EMS or Faradic are commonly used.

Nerve muscle physiology

In order to understand the action of muscle stimulating currents, it is necessary to understand nerve–muscle function.

Skeletal muscle

Skeletal muscle is composed of long, thin, multi-nucleated cells called muscle fibres. These muscle fibres are composed of myofibrils separated by sarcoplasm, and have an outer membrane called the sarcolemma. Muscle fibres are grouped together to form muscle bundles, and many bundles make up the complete muscle. Under an electron microscope, light and dark bands can be seen along the length of the fibre; these are known as A and I bands and are composed of two types of protein (actin and myosin). The movement of these bands into each other constitutes muscle contraction.

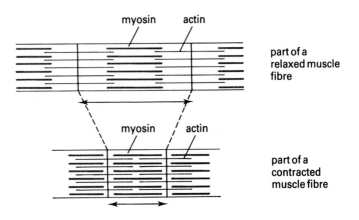

Figure 19.1 *Relaxed and contracted muscle fibres*

The contraction of skeletal muscle is controlled by the brain. Impulses initiated in the brain are transmitted via motor nerves to the muscle fibres, resulting in their contraction. Because the stimuli are electrical in nature, a suitable electrical pulse from a machine can be used to initiate a contraction. The electrical pulse can be applied anywhere along the course of a motor nerve, but the best response is obtained if it is applied at the point where the nerve enters the belly of the muscle, known as the *motor point.*

The nervous system

The system is made up of:

1 The central nervous system, comprising the *brain* and the *spinal cord.*

2 The peripheral nervous system comprising 12 pairs of *cranial* nerves (arising from the brain) and 31 pairs of *spinal* nerves (arising from the spinal cord).

3 The autonomic system.

Nervous tissue is composed of the functional units which conduct impulses called *neurones*, and the supporting tissue called *neuroglia*. There are three types of neurones:

1 *Sensory* neurones (or nerves): these carry impulses from the sensory organs to the spinal cord and brain.

2 *Motor* neurones: these carry impulses away from the brain and spinal cord to muscles and glands. These are the nerves stimulated by EMS.

3 *Connector* neurones or *interneurones*: these are found in the brain and spinal cord, and connect one group of neurones to another.

Neurones are similar in structure: they have a cell body and two types of processes called axons and dendrons.

- Axons carry impulses *away* from the cell body.
- Dendrons carry impulses *towards* the cell body.

Dendrons have small terminal branches called *dendrites*.

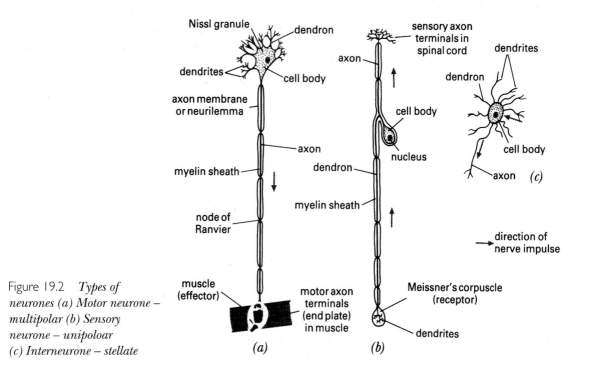

Figure 19.2   *Types of neurones (a) Motor neurone – multipolar (b) Sensory neurone – unipoloar (c) Interneurone – stellate*

The transmission of nerve impulses

Impulses are transmitted in axons and dendrons in one direction only. Impulses move along a nerve because of a change in its electrically charged state. This is brought about by the movement of positive and negative ions across the nerve membrane.

When the nerve membrane is at rest, solutions of sodium chloride, potassium chloride and various proteins are found inside and outside the membrane. The salts ionise in solution, giving sodium (+) ions and chloride (−) ions outside, with potassium (+) ions and chloride (−) ions inside, together with non diffusable anions, proteins inside the membrane which maintain the negative potential across the membrane.

When the nerve membrane is non-conductive, there are more positive ions outside and more negative ions inside. Therefore a potential difference exists across the membrane. In this state of rest the nerve is said to be *polarised.*

When a stimulus is applied to the nerve, the following reactions will occur: there will be a fall of potential difference across the membrane; the permeability of the membrane changes; the diffusable ions move across the membrane until the polarity is reversed – ie, there will be more negative ions outside and more positive ions inside. The nerve is now said to be *depolarised.*

When the concentration of ions reaches a certain level, the positive sodium ions are 'pumped out' and the nerve returns to its resting state, ie, is *re*polarised. This change of

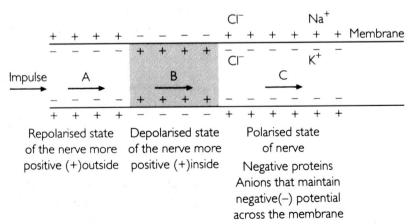

Figure 19.3 *Passage of a nerve impulse along an axon*

state occurs along the nerve and constitutes the passage of the impulse.

The impulse leaves A and is transmitted to B when the polarity reversed. The impulse will move along as the polarity returns to normal at B but reversed at C. The impulse is thus transmitted along the nerve fibre.

Synapse

More than one neurone will be involved in the transmission of a nerve impulse. Neurones do not connect directly with each other; there is always a gap between the end of one neurone and the beginning of another. This is known as a *synapse*. There are similarly specialised synapses between motor neurones and the muscle fibres they supply.

Pathway of an impulse

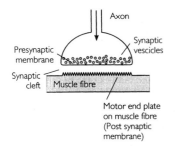

Figure 19.4 *Synapse between nerve terminal and muscle fibre*

An impulse initiated in the cells of the motor cortex of the brain will be transmitted via the axon (of the upper motor neurone) to the anterior/ventral horn of the spinal cord. Here the impulse will cross a synapse to stimulate the cell of another neurone (the lower motor neurone) to be transmitted via its axon to the muscle fibre.

Each anterior/ventral horn cell has one axon, which leaves the spinal cord by the anterior/ventral root. The axons of many cells will emerge together as a motor nerve and pass to a muscle where they will enter at the *motor point*. (When stimulating with an electrical pulse, the electrode should be placed over this point for maximum excitability.)

Each axon will then divide into many branches or terminals (from 5–150), depending on the function of the muscle. Muscles requiring fine control have smaller motor units with fewer branches, and can therefore produce more finely graded movements.

Each axon branch will supply one muscle fibre. The junction between the axon branch and the muscle fibre is known as the neuro-muscular junction. Here, the ends of the axons expand a little into bulbs; they approach but do not contact the muscle fibre. There is always a synapse in between. The sarcolemma covering the muscle fibre is modified at this point and is known as the motor end plate. The impulse is transmitted across the gap by the chemical transmitter acetylcholine.

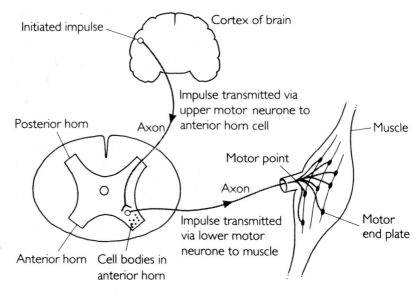

Figure 19.5 *Pathway of an impulse from the brain to a muscle fibre*

The anterior horn cell, the axon, axon branches and the muscle fibres they supply, make up the *motor unit*. This is not only an anatomical unit but also a functional unit. Impulses generated at the anterior horn cell will pass via the axon to all the fibres supplied by the axon branches, and all those fibres will contract simultaneously. The frequency of the impulses passing along the nerve will determine the strength of contraction in each motor unit.

During voluntary movement, motor units work an on/off 'shift' system; some will contract while others will be at rest. This allows fibres time to recover after contraction. When a stronger contraction is required, more motor units are activated. The frequency and number of motor units activated will determine the strength of contraction of the whole muscle.

With electrical stimulation, the frequency is usually selected at the beginning of the treatment and the strength of the contraction will depend on the density of current. An increase in current will stimulate more motor units and a stronger contraction will result.

Muscle fibre types

A muscle is composed of different types of muscle fibres. This enables individual muscles to perform various functions. Research has shown that these differences are imposed upon the fibres by their motor neurones. By imposing onto the fibre a certain pattern of activity, different physiological and biochemical properties develop. All the muscle fibres supplied by one motor neurone have similar properties.

Impulses from the central nervous system (CNS) which stimulate the different muscle fibres are discharged at different frequencies (shown below).

- *Slow twitch, slow oxidative fibres (SO) or red fibres:* These fibres are slow to contract and relax as their motor neuron fires at low frequency. Impulses are transmitted to these fibres at frequencies of between 6 Hz and 15 Hz.
- *Fast twitch, fast glycolytic fibres (FG) or white fibres:* The motor neuron supplying these fibres fires at a higher frequency. Impulses are transmitted to these fibres at frequencies of between 30 Hz and 80 Hz.
- *Fast oxidative glycolytic fibres (FOG):* Impulses are transmitted to these fibres at frequencies between 20 Hz and 40 Hz.

A muscle will be composed of a mixture of fibres – the percentage of each fibre type will differ for each muscle and will depend on the function of the muscle. Research has shown that electrical stimulation can be used to change muscle properties.

If fast glycolytic muscle fibres are stimulated at frequencies between 6 Hz and 15 Hz on a daily basis for a considerable length of time, they contract more slowly and do not fatigue easily. The biochemical characteristics are also changed; there is a decrease in glycolytic enzymes and an increase in oxidative enzymes; capillary density also increases. Thus, fast glycolytic fibres can be changed to slow oxidative fibres. (SO fibres do not seem to respond in the same way.)

This ability to change muscle fibre type is used medically in muscle transplant when the muscle is required to change its function; eg, replacing sphincters and cardiac assistance in heart disease.

Electrical stimulation machines

Modern machines which produce these pulses are very sophisticated electronic units: the older Faradic current has now largely been replaced by interrupted direct current.

Some non-British units use modified AC, but British units mainly use modified DC. These units produce low frequency, interrupted direct current between 10 Hz and 120 Hz. There are units on the market which offer upper range low frequency between 200 Hz and 800 Hz. Research has shown however that maximal force is developed in human muscle at between 40 Hz and 80 Hz. There is therefore little purpose in using higher frequencies, and careful consideration should be given to the effects of using these frequencies. Although sensory stimulation is reduced by higher frequencies, and they 'feel more comfortable', their safety and some of the claims made should be questioned as the mode in which they work is unclear.

Although there are a large number of different units available, one basic concept remains common to all – impulses are produced which stimulate the motor nerves resulting in the contraction of muscles supplied by those nerves. The muscles are made to contract actively and then relax, improving their tone and condition and maintaining strength, providing that the treatment is carried out on a regular basis.

Pulses, impulses and stimuli

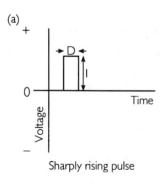

(a)

Sharply rising pulse

- The direct current must be modified to produce pulses which rise steeply and fall at regular intervals.
- A constant flow of current or a slow rising pulse will not produce a contraction, as the muscle adapts to the current; this is known as accommodation.
- The intensity must be high enough and duration of the pulse long enough to produce a contraction.
- I is the intensity of the current. On the machine, this is controlled by the intensity control to each pair of electrodes.
- D is the duration of the pulse or pulse width. This is pre-

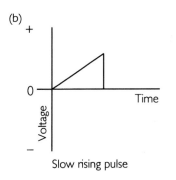

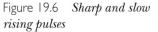

Slow rising pulse

Figure 19.6 *Sharp and slow rising pulses*

set on some machines but others have a pulse width control. A pulse width of under 100 μs is not effective and the best results are obtained with pulse widths of between 200 μs to 300 μs.

■ Some machines produce pulses of different shapes.
■ The shape of the pulse is known as the wave form.
■ It is the rate of rise of each pulse that determines the response in the muscle. A pulse which rises sharply produces the best response in innervated muscle and the rectangular pulse is generally used.
■ The number of pulses produced every second is known as the frequency and is measured in Hz.

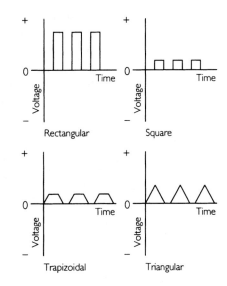

Figure 19.7 *Pulses of different shapes*

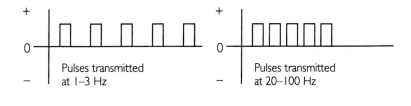

Pulses transmitted at 1–3 Hz

Pulses transmitted at 20–100 Hz

These pulses with a long interval in between allow the muscle to relax, thus producing a series of twitches

These pulses with short intervals in between do not allow the muscle to relax, thus producing a smooth fused contraction

Figure 19.8 *Pulses of different frequencies*

Tetanic contraction

A single adequate pulse will produce a twitch in the muscle. The muscle fibres contract as the current rises, and the contraction diminishes as the current falls; the muscle relaxes completely when the current stops.

- If a number of pulses are applied to the muscle, the type of contraction produced will depend on the interval between the pulses.
- If the interval between pulses is long enough for the fibres to relax, then a series of twitches will be produced in the muscle giving a tremulous contraction.
- If the pulses follow each other in rapid succession (ie, more pulses per second (higher frequency)), the muscle has no time to relax and a smooth contraction is produced. A smooth contraction of a muscle is known as a *tetanic* contraction.

Frequency

Frequency

20 Hz

Only slow fibres show fused contractions and the muscle contraction is not smooth

40 Hz

The majority of fibres show fused contractions and the muscle contraction becomes smoother

60 Hz

All fibres showing smooth, fused contraction and the muscle contraction is very smooth

Figure 19.9 *Muscle contraction at different frequency*

The frequency of the pulses is an important consideration because the different fibres within a muscle will respond in a different way to various frequencies:

- Below 20 Hz (ie, pulses per second), only the slow fibres will be showing smooth fused tetanic contractions; the faster fibres will be showing unfused contractions.
- As the frequency is increased to 40 Hz, the majority of fibres will be showing fused tetanic contractions, although some fast fibres may require higher frequencies to produce maximum force.
- At 60 Hz, the majority of fast fibres will be showing smooth fused tetanic contractions and the whole muscle will contract smoothly.

In most human muscle, maximal force is developed in the frequency range of 40–80 Hz and there is nothing to be gained by using higher frequencies. The highest frequency recorded during normal transmission is around 100 Hz.

Contraction time

The pulses are grouped together in 'trains' or 'envelopes' with rest period in between. When the current flows, the

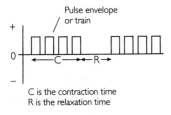

Pulse envelope or train

C is the contraction time
R is the relaxation time

Figure 19.10 *Trains or envelopes of pulses*

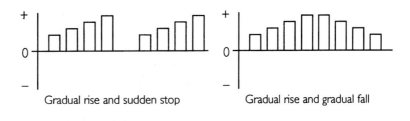

Gradual rise and sudden stop Gradual rise and gradual fall

Figure 19.11 *Surged envelopes*

muscle contracts; when the current stops, the muscle relaxes. This is similar to voluntary movement.

- On most machines, the contraction and relaxation period can be varied.
- In order to improve client comfort, the pulse envelope is surged so that the strength of the pulses rises gradually to peak intensity.
- The current may then stop suddenly on some units or decrease gradually on others.

- The rate of rise of the current is known as the *ramp* time.

Phasic selection

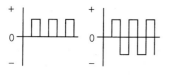

Monophasic–all the pulses are in one direction Biphasic–alternate pulses are reversed

Figure 19.12 *Monophasic and Biphasic pulses*

Many units have a phasic control and offer a choice of monophasic or biphasic current.

- With *monophasic*, the current flows mainly in one direction; ie, electrons flow from the negative electrode to the positive electrode without variation. Consequently the negative electrode (the cathode) will produce the stronger contraction. This is an important consideration when stimulating individual muscles, when the negative electrode (cathode) is placed over the motor point and the positive electrode (anode) is placed elsewhere.
- With *biphasic* current, each alternate pulse is reversed so that with the first pulse, electron flow is from cathode to anode, but the second pulse flow is reversed. In this way polarity is cancelled out and even strength contractions are produced under each pad. Either electrode can therefore be placed on the motor point.

Machine controls

Simple portable machines have few controls – usually an on/off switch, an intensity control, only one pair of pads, and perhaps a frequency control. The parameters would be preset and the only variable is the intensity control. They are usually used for the stimulation of individual muscles.

You may find large sophisticated machines in the clinic which have a range of variable controls and multi outlets for many pairs of pads. These can be used for stimulating single muscles, muscle groups or for general body padding. (It is important to have a complete understanding of the machine you are using; read the manufacturer's instructions thoroughly.) The machine may have some or all of the following controls.

On/off switch

This switches the current on and off. There is usually a light which comes on to show that the current is flowing.

Surge control/surge envelope/contraction time

This controls the length of time the current is flowing, ie, the length of the surge envelope or train. It therefore controls the length of the muscle contraction. While the current flows, the muscle will contract; when the current stops, the muscle relaxes. The surge length should be long enough to produce a good contraction. Muscles with poor tone or with a layer of covering fat require a longer surge.

The surge control usually varies from half a second to two and a half seconds.

C is the length of the contraction (contraction time)
R is the length of the relaxation (relaxation time)

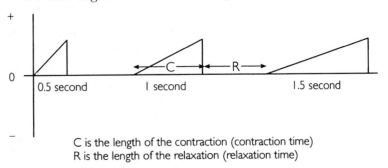

Figure 19.13 *Electronic surges of different length*

C is the length of the contraction (contraction time)
R is the length of the relaxation (relaxation time)

Relaxation control/interval or rest period

This controls the length of the rest period between the contractions. The rest period should be just longer than the surge period. This allows the muscle to relax fully, preventing muscle fatigue and build up of lactic acid which would cause pain and stiffness. It should not be too long. Many modern machines have an in-built automatic optimum relaxation time.

Ramp-time

This controls the rate of rise of the current in each surge; individual pulses are inhibited and gradually rise to build up to peak flow. Sharp rises give the best response. The rate must not be too slow as the muscle will accommodate.

Frequency control/pulses per second/Hz

This controls the number of pulses per second. Frequency determines the strength of contraction at the motor unit. Different fibre types will respond differently to different frequencies (see above). Therefore, by selecting a frequency of 40 Hz–60 Hz, most fibres in the muscle will be contracting smoothly.

The frequency within this range can be selected to provide the most comfortable smooth contraction for the client. If there is a tremor in the muscle, a higher frequency is needed.

Phase control (wave form)

This offers monophasic or biphasic pulses.

1 *Monophasic/Uniphasic/Single:* the current flows mainly in one direction, therefore the polarity of the pads remains the same for each contraction. One will be negative (the cathode) and the other positive (the anode). Leads usually indicate this by being colour-coded, or one having a groove or being rounded. Check with the manufacturer's instructions to establish which is which. When stimulating individual muscles, the cathode should always be placed on the motor point of the muscle as it produces the greatest response, while the anode is placed over another suitable area.
2 *Biphasic/Dual:* the current behaves like AC as alternate pulses are reversed, and it therefore eliminates polarity. It provides an even current under both pads, and either may be placed over the motor point.

Mode control/programme control

This controls the rhythms of the contraction and relaxation times.

1 *Constant:* the rhythm of the programme remains the same, once selected. The length of surge and interval remains the same throughout treatment.
2 *Variable/Rhythmic Active:* the rhythm of the surge and interval varies throughout the treatment. This has the advantage of preventing the client anticipating the contraction and resisting it. It is useful with tense, nervous clients. In many modern machines, a selection of variable contraction times will give the muscles thorough non-repetitious exercise.

Pulse width

This alters the width of each pulse. When pulse width is increased, it has a similar effect to increasing the intensity control. This is because additional current is provided because it is on for a longer period. Pulse widths under 100 µs are not effective; over 300 µs can be uncomfortable. Select 150–200 µs at commencement of treatment, and if the client cannot tolerate an increase in intensity due to discomfort, increasing the pulse width may produce a better contraction.

Maximum and minimum gain/master output

This increases current to all outlets together. It is used to increase intensity when client has become used to sensation. This control can be at zero at commencement of treatment, or it can be set midway so that the intensity can be increased or decreased during treatment.

Intensity controls (output controls)

These control the current flowing through each pair of pads. Most machines have an intensity control for one pair of pads. However there are machines where two pairs of pads share the same intensity control.

As the intensity control is turned up, the amount of current flowing through the pad increases.

■ When selecting intensity the best guide will be 'a good visible contraction within the tolerance of the client'.

Avoid turning the intensity too high, thinking that a stronger contraction is always better. Muscle fibres obey the 'all or none law', ie, once the stimulus is great enough to produce a contraction, there will be no increase in response of contracting fibres by turning up intensity. However, as the intensity of the current is increased, the strength of contraction is seen to increase (because more motor units are stimulated). Increasing the intensity will stimulate more motor units and therefore increase the strength of the contraction. Some machines have numbers around the intensity control which serve as a rough guide only. The intensity control will be turned up to obtain optimum maximum contraction with minimum discomfort.

Types of electrodes

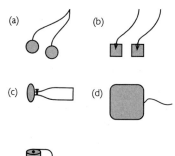

Figure 19.14 *Different electrodes*

The current is conducted from the machine to the client by means of leads and electrodes. These electrodes come in various forms:

1 *Rubber Pads:* these are the most common form of electrode. They are made of rubber impregnated with a good conductor such as graphite. They come in various sizes and may be round or square. Only one side is conductive, the other side is rubber insulated. They are held in place with strapping.
2 *Metal plates:* these are not usually found with modern equipment. They are made of tin, cut to the required size and attached to the lead with a clip. They are placed on top of 16 layers of lint and strapped to the part. Rubber strapping or crepe bandage may be used, but this must not get wet as it will become conductive. Place a non-absorbent layer such as rubber sheet over the lint before applying the bandage.
3 *Mushroom or disc electrode:* these are metal discs on the end of wooden handles. The discs are covered with 16 layers of lint. They are useful for individual stimulation of small muscles.
4 *Adhesive electrodes:* these are flexible rubberised pads impregnated with a good conductor. They have an adhesive on the conductive side and insulation on the other. They are placed over the appropriate areas and pressed onto the skin. They do not require strapping.
5 *Roller electrodes:* These are small metal cylinders covered with lint. They are used for labile treatments on large

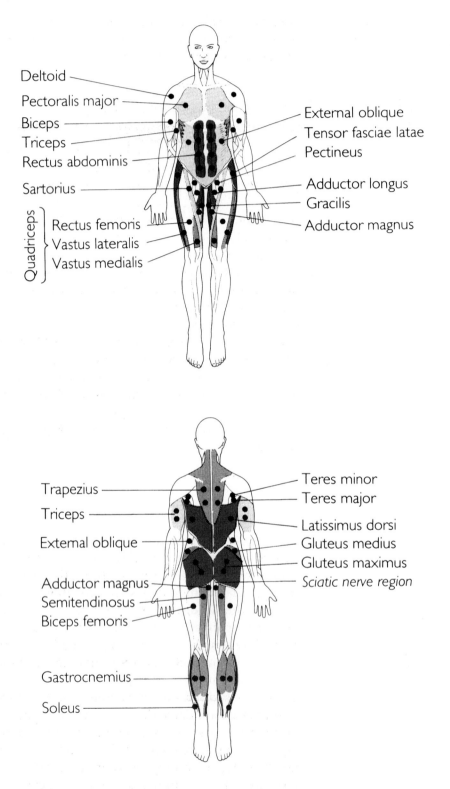

Deltoid
Pectoralis major
Biceps
Triceps
Rectus abdominis
Sartorius
Quadriceps
Rectus femoris
Vastus lateralis
Vastus medialis

External oblique
Tensor fasciae latae
Pectineus
Adductor longus
Gracilis
Adductor magnus

Trapezius
Triceps
External oblique
Adductor magnus
Semitendinosus
Biceps femoris
Gastrocnemius
Soleus

Teres minor
Teres major
Latissimus dorsi
Gluteus medius
Gluteus maximus
Sciatic nerve region

Figure 19.15   *Skeletal muscles and motor points (a) anterior (b) posterior*

sheets of muscle such as the back muscles. The roller is moved slowly over the back, stimulating the muscles as it passes over the motor points.

Physiological effects of electrical stimulation

1 Motor nerves are stimulated, resulting in muscle contraction. Selection of appropriate frequency will produce contraction of most fibres of a muscle. (This differs from active movement when only a percentage of fibres contract.) Increasing the intensity of the current will stimulate more motor units and increase the strength of the contraction.
2 The circulation is improved due to the pumping action of the contracting muscles. This increases the nutrients and oxygen brought to the part, and speeds up removal of waste products.
3 The metabolic rate of the cells is increased, which improves the condition of the muscle.
4 Nerve–muscle response is re-established following injury.
5 Stimulation of sensory nerves, giving the prickling sensation.
6 Superficial vasodilation and erythema is produced under the pads.

Uses

1 To improve the condition and strength of a muscle when combined with exercises. EMS may be combined with progressive resisted exercise in the early stages of strength training if muscles are weak, but phased out as strength develops. The same routine should be applied to both sides of the body to maintain balance.
2 To maintain muscle activity and strength when normal voluntary muscle contraction is inhibited by pain or injury; eg, stimulating the quadriceps after a knee injury, the gastrocnemius after an achilles tendon injury, deltoid following a shoulder injury, or triceps following an elbow injury. EMS must not be given immediately following injury, in the acute phase or if there is any risk of bleeding. It should only be given under medical direction, after accurate diagnosis. Isometric exercises should follow the treatment, progressing to isotonic as

strength develops.

3 To re-educate muscles following a period of immobility in plaster or strapping. Muscle strength decreases rapidly during a period of immobilisation; 20–30% may be lost in the first weeks. Initially daily stimulation is recommended, beginning with low intensity current and increasing gradually. Static exercises should be performed immediately after stimulation as explained above.

4 To treat postural scoliosis, when the muscles on the convex side of the curve are stimulated. The electrical treatment is followed by corrective exercises.

5 EMS may be given under pressure to reduce oedema. This is achieved by placing the electrodes above and below the swelling, and then applying a crepe or rubber bandage to the whole area. The part is then elevated. The contraction of the muscles beneath the bandage has a squeezing effect, which aids absorption of the swelling.

Contra-indications

1 Acute muscle injury or spasm, acute ligament or tendon injuries, any risk of bleeding.

2 Broken bones.

3 Extensive cuts and bruises (small cuts may be insulated with petroleum jelly).

4 Skin infections, as there is a risk of spreading the condition.

5 Recent scar tissue, as it may break down.

6 Metal pins and plates such as pinned or plated fractures, as the current may concentrate here.

7 Pacemakers. Padding of the arms back and chest should be avoided as the frequency of electrical pulses can interfere with the pacemaker.

8 Heart conditions, as the increase in speed of circulation can impose stress on the heart.

9 High or low blood pressure (see above).

10 Thrombosis, as blood clots may become dislodged.

11 Phlebitis (see above).

12 Do not pad heavily in the chest region near the heart, as the current may interfere with nerve conduction to the heart.

Dangers

There are no specific dangers attached to EMS. Discomfort can be caused if the intensity is too high, if the pads are in the wrong position (ie, not on motor points), if the pads are too close to or over bony points, or if there are any open abrasions that are not insulated (the current will concentrate here).

- Muscle fatigue can be produced if the intensity is too high, if the rest interval is too short or treatment is prolonged.
- An initial sudden surge of current will feel like a shock, therefore it is important to turn up during the surge so that the client can feel intensity increasing gradually. Turn off during rest period.
- Heavy padding of the chest region should be avoided as stimuli may interfere with heart rhythm.

Precautions

Figure 19.16 *Padding for individual muscles (a) Rectus femoris (b) Rectus femoris and vastus medialis (c) Vastus medialis and vastus lateralis (d) Deltoid*

1 When intensity is turned up *never* move pads, press pads down or push terminals in.
2 Check for contra-indications.
3 Test the machine.

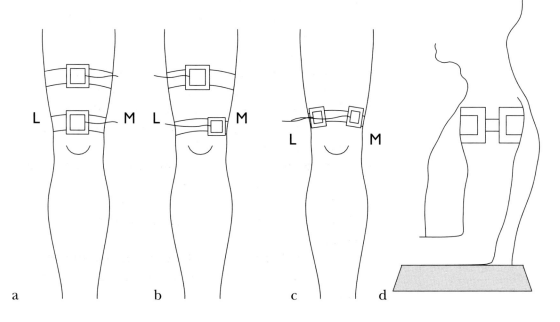

a   b   c   d

4 Select appropriate points on all controls.
5 Ensure intensity controls are at zero before increasing intensity.
6 Check pads and wet with saline or water.
7 Strap pads securely with even pressure.
8 Check outlets before switching on.
9 Turn *up* during *surge* only.
10 Avoid heavy padding of chest region; pad anterior or posterior but not both.

The stimulation of individual muscles

The sports therapist may be required to stimulate individual muscles or specific muscle groups, depending on the condition being treated.

Padding

Firstly check whether the machine offers both biphasic and monophasic current.

■ When stimulating individual muscles with one motor point, monophasic is the usual choice. The stronger cathode is the active electrode and is placed on the motor point; the indifferent electrode (the anode) is placed proximal to it. Simple machines may not identify polarity, in which case the current is probably biphasic.
  If the machine produces biphasic current only, the current under each pad will be equal if the pads are of equal size. To produce a stronger effect at the active electrode, the density of current under this electrode must be increased. This is achieved by making the active electrode smaller than the indifferent, but of course this is not always possible, as rubber electrodes are usually of equal size.
■ When stimulating long muscles with two motor points, a pad is placed on each point and the current may be mono or biphasic.
■ When stimulating small muscles, a disc electrode may be used as the active electrode (cathode), which is held in

place on the motor point of the muscle, and a larger plate electrode is strapped, proximal and nearby.

▪ When stimulating two muscles such as vastus medialis and vastus lateralis, the pads will be placed on the motor points of each muscle. If the current is monophasic, the cathode should be placed on vastus medialis or the weaker muscle.

Treatment technique

Decide on the appropriate method of padding. As explained above, the current is applied to each muscle or group using two electrodes. One electrode known as the active electrode is placed on the motor point of the muscle; the other known as the indifferent is placed nearby, usually proximal to the active.

The electrodes may be two rubber electrodes strapped to the part, or two metal electrodes placed over sixteen layers of lint and held in place by rubber strapping or two adhesive electrodes which are pressed over the motor point.

Preparation of the client

1 Place the client in a well supported, comfortable position with the muscle to be treated in its shortened position. Ensure that there is no tight clothing restricting muscle action, eg, tight shorts around the quadriceps or tight sleeves around triceps.
2 Check that there is no metal in the area, eg, chains, rings, jewellery etc.
3 Clean the area thoroughly to remove dirt and sebum; use wipes or soap and water; rinse and dry.
4 Check for contra-indications.
5 Examine the part for any small cuts or abrasions. Cover these with petroleum jelly and plaster.
6 Explain the treatment to the client, ie, a prickling sensation, then a contraction.
7 Ask the client to report any discomfort during the treatment.
8 Pre-heating the area will increase the response. Any suitable or available method may be used providing there are no contra-indications to heat.

Procedure

1 Place the machine on a suitable stable base and check that the plugs, pads and leads are secure.
2 Collect all commodities such as hot water or saline solution, cologne, lint, cotton.
3 Clean the skin and check for cuts; cover these with petroleum jelly or plaster.
4 Check that the intensity controls are at zero and switch the machine on.
5 Check the machine on yourself.
6 Moisten the surface of the pads, or if using metal electrodes, wet the lint with saline and fold into 16 layers, sides to middle. Place the lint between the skin and the electrode.
7 Identify the muscle to be treated and its motor point. Place and strap the active electrode over the motor point; if using monophasic current, this will be the cathode. Place the inactive electrode proximal to it, on a convenient area nearby, strap firmly to ensure a firm even contact between skin and electrodes.
8 Select the appropriate controls.
9 Turn the intensity control up slowly until a good visible contraction is obtained, which must be within the tolerance of the client.
10 The intensity may be increased after a time, as the client becomes used to the treatment and the pads dry out.
11 Treat for 20–30 minutes. Switch off.
12 Turn the intensity control back to zero.
13 Remove the electrodes and strapping.
14 Dry the area thoroughly.
15 Clean the pads with warm water and detergent.
16 Follow with appropriate exercises and teach home exercises.

Reasons for poor contractions

1 The intensity is too low.
2 The pads are too dry or dirty.
3 The pads are off the motor points or near tendons.
4 Poor contact between pads and skin.
5 Poor contact at leads and terminals.
6 Treating over a depth of fat.

Questions

1 Describe the composition of skeletal muscle.
2 List the parts of the nervous system.
3 Define the following
   A motor point
   B neuro-muscular junction
   C motor end plate
   D motor unit
4 List three types of muscle fibres and give the transmission frequencies to produce smooth contractions of each fibre type.
5 Why should the electrodes/pads be placed on the motor point of a muscle.
6 Give three reasons for use of individual muscle stimulation.
7 Explain four physiological effects of EMS.
8 Explain the purpose of the following controls found on machines.

   A intensity control
   B surge length
   C relaxation length
   D phasic control
   E pulse width
   F maximum/minimum gain or master control
   G rhythm control

9 Strength of contraction is not only governed by the intensity of the current, list six other factors which influence the strength of contractions.
10 List six contra-indications to the stimulation of individual or superficial body muscles.
11 Describe four factors which may result in poor contractions.
12 Explain why the cathode should be the active electrode when stimulating individual muscles using monophasic current.

Further reading

Alter, M. J. (1988) *Science of Stretching*, Human Kinetics Book.

Bean, Anita (second edn) *The Complete Guide to Sports Nutrition*, A and C Black, London.

Beashel and Taylor (1996) *Physical Education and Sport*, Nelson.

Egger, G. and Champion, N. (1990) *The Fitness Leaders Handbook*, Kangaroo Press.

Grisogono, Vivian (1989) *Sports Injuries*, Churchill Livingstone.

Harris, Lovesey and Oram (1982) *The Sports Health Handbook*, The Kingswood Press.

Hayes, Fiona (1995) *Fitness Programming*, Summit.

Jenson and Schults (1970) *Applied Kinesiology*, McGraw-Hill Book Company.

Katch and McArdle (1993) *Introduction to Nutrition, Exercise and Health*, Lea and Febiger.

McLatchie, G. R. (1993) *Essentials of Sports Medicine*, Churchill Livingstone.

Peterson and Renstrom (1993) *Sports Injuries, their Prevention and Treatment*, Martin Dunitz Ltd.

Tortora, Gerard J. (1991) *Introduction to the Human Body*, Harper Collins.

Index

abrasions   269
acceleration   85
active movement   112
active stretch   21
adenosine triphosphate   57
aerobic energy system   58
aerobic exercise   60
aerobic exercise classes   240
agonists   106
alactate system   57
all or none law   53
amino acids   69
anaerobic energy system   57
anaerobic exercise   60
analysis of muscle work   108
anatomical position   26
angular/rotary motion   89
antagonists   106
antigravity muscles   93
antioxidants   75
aponeuroses   54
appendicular skeleton   31
application of forces   86
asthma   19
axes of movement   43
axial skeleton   31

base   94
basal metabolic rate   63
blisters   269
body composition   80
body mass index   81
bones of the skeletal system   30–5
bone structure   29
breathing exercises   215
breathing mechanism   40

calcium   72
calories   62
carbohydrates   63
    disaccharides   64
    monosaccharides   64
    polysaccharides   64
    simple/complex   64
cardio-respiratory endurance   120–7
care and safety of equipment   10
cartilaginous joint   44
cell structure   14
centre of gravity   93
chemical levels   13
cholesterol   23, 68
choreography   241
circuit training   125, 132
class preparation   237
classification of movement   111
client safety and hygiene   7, 9
clothing and footwear   7
codes of practice   2
common injuries   275–85
components of fitness   118

concentric work   104
conditioning phase   122, 237
contra-indications to exercise   11
contusions   269
cool down exercises   213, 237
cross training   125
cryotherapy (ice therapy)   286–94
    contra-indications   289
    exercises after ice treatment   293
    methods of application   286
    physiological effects   287
    rate of cooling   289
    treatment techniques   290–3
    uses   289
cuts   269

damaging effects of inappropriate
    exercise   24
damaging exercises   216–27
dehydration   76
diabetes   24
diet   62–83
direction   84

eccentric work   104
ectomorph   81
effects of exercise, on   13
    bones   21
    cardio-vascular system   18
    connective tissue structures   21
    joints   21
    metabolism   22
    neuromuscular coordination   22
    respiratory system   18
    skeletal muscle   19
electrical muscle stimulation   336–59
    contraction time   346
    contra-indications   354
    dangers   355
    frequency   346
    machines   344
    machine controls   347–51
    motor points of skeletal muscles   352
    muscle fibre types   342
    nerve-muscle physiology   337–42
    padding   356
    physiological effects   353
    precautions   355
    pulses/stimuli   344
    reasons for poor contractions   358
    terminology   337
    tetanic contraction   346
    treatment technique   357
    types of electrodes   351
    uses   353
endomorph   81
endurance training   120
endurance training
    effects/precautions   125–6
energy   62

energy nutrients   63
ethical standards   2

fats   66
fartlek running   124
feedback   233
fibre intake   79
fibrous joint   44
first aid   262
fitness assessment   247
    blood pressure test   258
    body composition   256
    body measurement   249
    client preparation   247
    consent form   248
    flexibility test   259
    grip test   252
    height measurement   249
    lung capacity test   257
    muscle strength   251
    muscle tone   252–4
    step test   254
    weight measurement   249
fitness training   114
fixators   106, 107
flat back   197
flexibility   157–75
    effects   163
    factors affecting   157
    methods of increasing   159–63
force   85, 86
fractures   273
free radicals   74
functions of the skeletal system   27

general benefits of exercise   22
glucose   64
gravity   92
    anti-gravity muscles   93
    centre of   93
    line of   94
group action of muscles   106

healthy eating   82
heart disease   24
heat therapy   295–326
    contra-indications to heat   295
    methods   295
homeostasis   14
hypertension   24

impetus   85
inertia   85
infections   269
infra red treatment   296
    contra-indications   304
    dangers   304
    effects of infra red   300–3
    heat after injury   306
    intensity of radiation   298–300
    lamps   296–8

infra red treatment – *cont.*
  precautions   305
  treatment technique   305
  uses of infra red   303
injuries   268
injury assessment   263
inter-vertebral discs   37
iron   73
isokinetic training   131
isometric muscle work   105
isometric strength training   129
isotonic muscle work   103
isotonic strength training   130

joints   41–9
joint movement   41–2
  classification   44
  features   47
  range   46
  terminology   41
joules   63

kyphosis   193
kypho-lordosis   194

lactate system   57
learning new skills   230
legislative requirements   2
levers   96
ligament injuries   271
linear/translatory motion   89
line of gravity   94
lipoproteins   23, 68
lordosis   190

magnitude   84
macrocycle   246
mass   84
maximum heart rate   121
macronutrients   63
mechanical massage   327–35
  gyratory vibrator   328
    contra-indications   330
    dangers   331
    effects   329
    precautions   331
    treatment technique   332
  audio-sonic vibrator   333
    contra-indications   334
    effects   332
    uses   334
    treatment technique   334
megacycle   246
mesocycle   246
mesomorph   81
metabolism   22
microcycle   246
micronutrients   63
minerals   72
mobility exercises   205–11
momentum   85
motion   89
motivation   232
muscle attachments   54
muscle contraction   56
muscle diagrams   50–1
muscle endurance   20
muscle endurance training   136
muscle fatigue   61
muscle fibres   51
muscle fitness   127
muscle injuries   270
muscle strength/bulk   19
muscle strength training   131–5
muscle structure   51
muscle tone   56

neuromuscular coordination   22

Newton's Laws of Motion   90–2
nutrition   62–83

objectives   235
oesteoporosis   21
organs   16
organisational levels   13
oxygen debt   60
oxygen uptake   59

paraffin wax treatment   323
  care of wax   326
  contra-indications   325
  dangers   325
  effects   324
  equipment   324
  precautions   325
  treatment technique   325
  uses   324
passive movement   112
passive stretch   21
pelvic girdle   38
periodised training   246
personal safety and hygiene   5
phosphocreatine   57
physical principles   85
physiological benefits of exercise   23
phytochemicals   63, 75
planes of movement   43
planning for individual exercise   244
planning exercise classes   234
planning exercises to music   242
plyometrics   137
posture   183–99
  correction   189
  effects of good/bad posture   183
  evaluation   185
postural problems and their
    correction   190
prevention of injury   262
programme planning   245
proteins   68
psychological benefits of exercise   24

range of movement   105
reasons for stopping exercising   239
relationships with clients   4
relationships with colleagues   3
relaxation   176–82
  aids   177
  preparation   178
  techniques   179
response to exercise   18
rest   176
ribs   40
'RICED'   264
round shoulders   195
running   123

safety
  and hygiene   5
  of clients   9
  of premises   8
  when using equipment   10
sauna baths   311
  contra-indications   313
  dangers   313
  differences between steam/sauna   315
  effects   313
  precautions   314
  treatment technique   314
  uses   313
scalar quantity   84
selecting music   241
setting objectives/goals   235
sequence of activities   236
shoulder girdle   38
skeletal muscle   50–61

skeletal system   27–49
  bones   30
  features of skeletal bones   32–5
  functions   27
skill   229
slipped disc   37
spa pools/baths   315
  contra-indications   319
  dangers   319
  effects   318
  installation   316
  operation and care   320
  operator responsibilities   320
  precautions   319
  preparation of client   323
  protection of operator   322
  purification   317
  uses   318
  water standards   317
speed   85, 153
spinal column   35
spinal curves   36
spinal problems   36
sports drinks   77–9
stability   95
starting positions   201
steam treatments   307–11
  contra-indications   309
  dangers   309
  effects of steam heat   308
  precautions   310
  steam baths/room   306
  treatment technique   311
  uses of steam heat   309
sternum   39
strengthening exercises   138–53
stretching exercises   164–75, 236
structure of bone   29
suppleness   157
surface terminology   27
  anterior/posterior   27
  medial/lateral   27
  proximal/distal   27
  superficial/deep   27
  superior/inferior   27
synergists   107
synovial joint   44–6
systems of the body   16

target heart rate   122
teaching exercises   228
tendon injuries   271
thoracic cavity   39
tissues   15
treatments   261
treatment of soft tissue injuries   273
training principles   116
  duration   117
  frequency   117
  intensity   117
  overload   117
  progression   117
  specificity   116
  training threshold   116

vector   84
velocity   85
vertebra   37
vertebral column   35
vertebral discs   37
vitamins   70
VO maximum   59

warm up exercises   212, 236
water intake   75
weight   84
weight control   79
winged scapulae   199